Handbook of
Endocrine Protocols

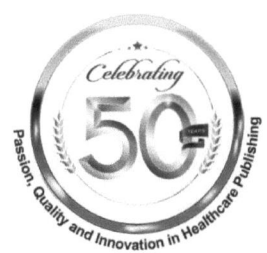

Handbook of Endocrine Protocols

Second Edition

Simon Rajaratnam
MBBS MD DNB (Endo) MNAMS FRACP (Endo) PhD (Endo) FRCP (Edin)
Head
Department of Endocrinology, Diabetes and Metabolism
Christian Medical College
Vellore, Tamil Nadu, India

Anulekha Mary John
MBBS MD Fellowship (Endo)
Endocrinologist and Associate Professor
Believers Church Medical College Hospital
Thiruvalla, Kerala, India

Foreword
Nihal Thomas

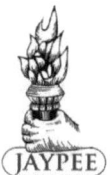

JAYPEE BROTHERS MEDICAL PUBLISHERS
The Health Sciences Publisher
New Delhi | London | Panama

Jaypee Brothers Medical Publishers (P) Ltd.

Headquarters
Jaypee Brothers Medical Publishers (P) Ltd
4838/24, Ansari Road, Daryaganj
New Delhi 110 002, India
Phone: +91-11-43574357
Fax: +91-11-43574314
Email: jaypee@jaypeebrothers.com

Overseas Offices

J.P. Medical Ltd
83 Victoria Street, London
SW1H 0HW (UK)
Phone: +44 20 3170 8910
Fax: +44 (0)20 3008 6180
Email: info@jpmedpub.com

Jaypee-Highlights Medical Publishers Inc
City of Knowledge, Bld. 235, 2nd Floor
Clayton, Panama City, Panama
Phone: +1 507-301-0496
Fax: +1 507-301-0499
Email: cservice@jphmedical.com

Jaypee Brothers Medical Publishers (P) Ltd
Bhotahity, Kathmandu, Nepal
Phone: +977-9741283608
Email: kathmandu@jaypeebrothers.com

Website: www.jaypeebrothers.com
Website: www.jaypeedigital.com

© 2019, Jaypee Brothers Medical Publishers

The views and opinions expressed in this book are solely those of the original contributor(s)/author(s) and do not necessarily represent those of editor(s) of the book.

All rights reserved. No part of this publication may be reproduced, stored or transmitted in any form or by any means, electronic, mechanical, photocopying, recording or otherwise, without the prior permission in writing of the publishers.

All brand names and product names used in this book are trade names, service marks, trademarks or registered trademarks of their respective owners. The publisher is not associated with any product or vendor mentioned in this book.

Medical knowledge and practice change constantly. This book is designed to provide accurate, authoritative information about the subject matter in question. However, readers are advised to check the most current information available on procedures included and check information from the manufacturer of each product to be administered, to verify the recommended dose, formula, method and duration of administration, adverse effects and contraindications. It is the responsibility of the practitioner to take all appropriate safety precautions. Neither the publisher nor the author(s)/editor(s) assume any liability for any injury and/or damage to persons or property arising from or related to use of material in this book.

This book is sold on the understanding that the publisher is not engaged in providing professional medical services. If such advice or services are required, the services of a competent medical professional should be sought.

Every effort has been made where necessary to contact holders of copyright to obtain permission to reproduce copyright material. If any have been inadvertently overlooked, the publisher will be pleased to make the necessary arrangements at the first opportunity. The **CD/DVD-ROM** (if any) provided in the sealed envelope with this book is complimentary and free of cost. **Not meant for sale.**

Inquiries for bulk sales may be solicited at: jaypee@jaypeebrothers.com

Handbook of Endocrine Protocols

First Edition: 2015
Second Edition: **2019**

ISBN: 978-93-5270-698-3

Dedicated to

Our Alma mater
Christian Medical College, Vellore
Tamil Nadu, India

Foreword

The beginning of any good book is like the source of a river on top of a mountain. The view from there is magnificent, the water is clean and a cool-breeze kisses your skin as you gaze at the swirling ripples cascade down into the valley.

Akin to this allegory, is the opportunity that I have had when reviewing the contents of this book.

Just as a few thousand readers have had the chance to gain knowledge from this little mini-encyclopedia on endocrinology through the first edition; so may many thousands more refresh themselves in their few precious moments that follow the many hours of toil and work in their busy days as clinicians, thereby enabling them to fill in the missing links and gaps in their knowledge.

Having an approach and algorithm to medical disorders and diseases is extremely important to help in the development of a robust differential diagnosis and an accurate therapeutic plan.

With the increasing diversity of clinical endocrinology being supported by a rapidly growing armamentarium of diagnostic tests, the tendency for an experienced clinician is to assume that what has been known and is time tested is a foregone conclusion of being precise. However, knowledge needs updation to supplement experience-based wisdom.

Similarly, therapeutic agents have also undergone a certain degree of advancement and evolution. Their availability may vary from continent to continent. Taking this into account, the authors have spent many months in trying to modify chapters to suit the needs of the practicing physician in South Asia.

The wonder that one experiences when practicing clinical endocrinology is like that of a child taking a tour in a zoological park. This book only helps enhance our starry-eyed gazed of this beautiful science.

All-in-all Drs Simon Rajaratnam and Anulekha Mary John have burnt the midnight oil in manufacturing a top class product.

As our finger tips caress the margins of the pages, I am certain that pages will turn brown, through use and reuse, and like any book which stands the test of time as a classic, the binding may loosen as an indicator of excellence.

Once again I wish one and all: "Bonne Lecture!"

Nihal Thomas
MD MNAMS DNB (Endo) FRACP (Endo) FRCP (Edin)
FRCP (Glas) FRCP (London) PhD (Copenhagen)
Professor and Head, Unit-1
Department of Endocrinology, Diabetes and Metabolism
Associate Director
Christian Medical College
Vellore, Tamil Nadu, India

Preface to the Second Edition

What I love about Medicine is that it keeps constantly changing as new discoveries are made. To keep up-to-date with current literature we have had to revise and come up a new edition of this booklet. We have strived to keep it simple and user friendly. We have introduced a new tabular format for the testing protocols. Most of the diagnostic tests can be easily completed as a day-care. All the reference ranges mentioned in this booklet are taken from the Department of Clinical Biochemistry, Christian Medical College, Vellore, Tamil Nadu, India. These treatment protocols are for adult patients and they should never be extrapolated for the pediatric age group.

Simon Rajaratnam

Preface to the First Edition

From my experience both as a student and as a teacher I felt the need for a small handbook which will serve as a ready reckoner for those working in the field of Endocrinology. With this in mind I tried to simplify details and present information in a simple format.

The Biochemistry reference ranges mentioned in this book are taken from the Department of Clinical Biochemistry, Christian Medical College, Vellore, Tamil Nadu, India. The section on Endocrine Test Protocols is specifically written as to enable these tests being performed as Day Care, with all the patients coming in by 8 AM. The treatment protocols in this book are meant only for adult patients and these should not be extrapolated for pediatric patients.

I am grateful to my teacher Dr MS Seshadri who nurtured my career in Endocrinology. I would also like to acknowledge the contribution of my coauthor Dr Anulekha Mary John who has been my student. This knowledge continues to be passed on from one generation to another.

Simon Rajaratnam

Acknowledgments

A great teacher inspires his students and I am fortunate to have had Dr MS Seshadri as my mentor and my guide. I am also fortunate to have my former student Dr Anulekha Mary John as my co-author. We are all grateful to our Alma mater The Christian Medical College, Vellore, Tamil Nadu, India, for molding and making us what we are today.

I would like to thank Shri Jitendar P Vij (Group Chairman), Mr Ankit Vij (Managing Director), Ms Chetna Malhotra Vohra (Associate Director—Content Strategy) and the staff of M/s Jaypee Brothers Medical Publishers (P) Ltd., New Delhi, India.

Contents

Chapter 1. Clinical Biochemistry: Reference Ranges   1

Chapter 2. Evaluation of Endocrine Disorders   4

Chapter 3. Endocrine Test Protocols   11

Chapter 4. Treatment Protocols   31

Chapter 5. Endocrine Emergencies   37

Chapter 6. Diabetes Protocols   45

Chapter 7. Common Calculations and Scoring Systems   56

Chapter 8. Drug Doses   63

Index   *73*

CHAPTER 1

Clinical Biochemistry: Reference Ranges

RENAL PARAMETERS	
Sodium	135–145 mmol/L
Potassium	3.5–5 mmol/L
Bicarbonate	22–29 mmol/L
Chloride	95–105 mmol/L
Urea	15–40 mg/dL
Creatinine	0.7–1.4 mg/dL (males) 0.5–1.1 mg/dL (females)

BONE PROFILE	
Calcium	8.3–10.4 mg/dL
Albumin	3.5–5.0 g/dL
Phosphate	2.5–4.6 mg/dL
Alkaline phosphatase	40–125 U/L
Vitamin D (25 OHD$_3$)	>30 ng/mL
Parathyroid hormone	8–74 pg/mL
24-hr urinary calcium	50–300 mg/24 hr

LIPID PROFILE	
Total cholesterol	<200 mg/dL
Triglyceride	<150 mg/dL
LDL cholesterol	<100 mg/dL
HDL cholesterol	>60 mg/dL

LIVER FUNCTION TESTS (LFTs)	
Bilirubin total	0.5–1 mg/dL
Bilirubin direct	0.1–0.5 mg/dL
Protein	6.0–8.5 g/dL
Albumin	3.5–5.0 g/dL
Alanine amino-transferase (ALT or SGPT)	5–35 U/L
Aspartate amino transferase (AST or SGOT)	8–40 U/L
Alkaline phosphatase	40–125 U/L

DIABETES			
Glucose			
Fasting (AC)		Normal	<100 mg/dL
		Impaired fasting glucose	100–125 mg/dL
		Diabetes mellitus	≥126 mg/dL
2 hr postmeal (PC)		Normal	<140 mg/dL
		Impaired glucose tolerance	140–199 mg/dL

Contd...

Contd...

	Diabetes mellitus	≥200 mg/dL
HbA1c		
	Normal	<5.7%
	Prediabetes	5.7–6.4%
	Diabetes	≥6.5%
C-Peptide	1.1–5.0 ng/mL	
Antiglutamic acid decarboxylase (GAD) antibody	<5.0 U/mL	
Anti-islet cell antibody	<7.5 U/mL	
Insulin (fasting)	0–30 µU/mL	
Urine microalbumin	<30 mg/g creatinine	
Urine protein/creatinine	<0.21 mg/mg	
24-hr urine protein	50–150 mg/24-hr	

HORMONE ASSAYS

Thyroid

Total thyroxine (TT$_4$)	4.5–12.5 µg/dL			
Free thyroxine (FT$_4$)	0.8–2.0 ng/dL	*Gonadal hormones*		
Total T$_3$	90–190 ng/dL	Follicle stimulating hormone (FSH) (Women)		
Thyroid stimulating hormone (TSH)	0.3–4.5 mIU/L	Follicular phase	2.8–11.3 mIU/mL	
Thyroid antibodies -		Mid-cycle	5.8–21 mIU/mL	
Antimicrosomal (TPO) antibodies	<50 IU/mL	Luteal phase	1.2–9 mIU/mL	
Antithyroglobulin antibodies	<100 IU/mL	Postmenopausal	21.7–153 mIU/mL	
Thyroglobulin (Post-thyroidectomy)	<1 ng/mL	(Men)	0.7–11.1 mIU/mL	
Calcitonin	0–50 pg/mL			
		Luteinizing hormone (LH) (Women)		
Adrenal		Follicular phase	1.1–11.6 mIU/mL	
17 OH-progesterone		Mid-cycle	17–77 mIU/mL	
Men	0.4–3.3 ng/mL	Luteal phase	0.0–14.7 mIU/mL	
Women (Follicular phase)	0.1–1.2 ng/mL	Postmenopausal	11.3–39.8 mIU/mL	
(Luteal phase)	0.4–4.8 ng/mL	(Men)	0.8–7.6 mIU/mL	

Contd...

Contd...

Dehydroepiandrosterone sulfate (DHEAS)	
Men	80–560 µg/dL
Women	35–430 µg/dL
Plasma renin	2.8–39.9 µIU/mL

Aldosterone	
Supine	10–160 pg/mL
Upright	40–310 pg/mL
Urine metanephrine	<350 mg/day
Urine normetanephrine	<600 mg/day

Pituitary	
Human growth hormone (basal)	0–5.0 ng/mL
(1 hour postglucose)	<0.4 ng/mL
(2 hour postglucose)	<0.4 ng/mL
Insulin like growth factor-1 (IGF-1)	
10 years	88–452 ng/mL
20 years	127–424 ng/mL
26–30 years	117–329 ng/mL
46–50 years	94–252 ng/mL
66–70 years	69–200 ng/mL
Adreno corticotrophic hormone (ACTH)	0–46 pg/mL
Cortisol	
Basal (morning)	7–25 µg/dL
Post-Synacthen (30 and 60 min)	>20 µg/dL
Post-Dexa	<1.8 µg/dL
24-hr urinary free cortisol (UFC)	10–55 µg/24-hr

Estradiol	
Follicular phase	0–0.587 nmol/L
Luteal phase	0.1–0.91 nmol/L

Progesterone	
Follicular phase	1.00–3.80 nmol/L
Mid-cycle	1.70–50 nmol/L
Luteal Phase	2.30–56.60 nmol/L

Prolactin	
Women	1.9–25.0 ng/mL
Men	2.5–17 ng/mL

Testosterone	
Women	50–120 ng/dL
Men (20–49 yrs)	270–1030 ng/dL
(>50 yrs)	212–755 ng/dL

Sex hormone binding globulin (SHBG)	
Women	26.1–110 nmol/L
Men	14.5–48.4 nmol/L
Inhibin A	<97 pg/mL
Anti-Müllerian hormone (AMH)	2.0–6.8 ng/mL

CHAPTER 2

Evaluation of Endocrine Disorders

THYROID				
Basic tests			Additional tests	
	Total T$_4$			Total T$_3$
	Free T$_4$			Free T$_3$
	TSH			Thyroid antibodies*
				TSH receptor antibodies**
Imaging			* For patients with suspected thyroiditis	
	Ultrasound (US) neck		**For patients with Graves' disease	
	I^{131} uptake scan			
	Technetium (Tc) scan			

THYROID MALIGNANCY				
Tests	Fine needle aspiration cytology (FNAC)		On follow-up check	
	Calcitonin			Total T$_4$ and Free T$_4$
	Thyroglobulin			Calcium
	Antithyroglobulin antibodies			Phosphate
	Carcinoembryonic antigen (CEA)			Albumin
	Biopsy report with tumor staging			
	I^{131} whole body scan			
	Ultrasound (US) neck			
	Computed tomography (CT) scan			
	Positron emission tomography (PET) scan			

Evaluation of Endocrine Disorders

PARATHYROID				
Basic tests			Additional tests	
	Calcium			24-hour urinary calcium, phosphorus and creatinine
	Phosphorus			Calculate $FePO_4$ and Tmp/GFR
	Albumin			Screen for other associated endocrine tumors involving the pituitary and pancreas • Prolactin, HGH • Fasting blood sugar and insulin (Insulinoma) • Glucagon (Glucagonoma)
	Alkaline phosphatase			
	Vitamin D			
	Parathyroid hormone (PTH)			
	Magnesium			
Imaging				
	Sestamibi scan with SPECT-CT			
	US neck			
	Kidney urinary bladder (KUB) X-ray			
	Bone density			

PANCREAS		
Suspected insulinoma	72-hour fasting test	
Imaging		
	CT scan/magnetic resonance imaging (MRI)	
	Endoscopic ultrasound	
	68Ga-DOTATATE PET scan	

DIABETES MELLITUS			
Basic tests	Fasting blood sugar (AC)	Additional tests	Electrolytes
	Postprandial blood sugar (PC)		Urine ketones
	Hemoglobin A1c (HbA1c)		Blood gas
	Lipid profile		Vitamin B_{12}
	Creatinine		
	A : G ratio		
	Urine—microalbumin		
	Urine—protein/creatinine ratio		
	Electrocardiogram (ECG)		
	Ophthalmic evaluation		

Contd...

Contd...

		C-peptide	MODY	Genetic studies
Type–1 diabetes		Glutamic acid decarboxylase (GAD) antibodies		
		Anti-islet cell antibodies	Gestational diabetes	Oral glucose tolerance test (OGTT)
Screening for other associated disorders		TSH, thyroid antibodies		Fasting blood sugar (AC)
		Calcium, phosphorus, albumin, alkaline phosphatase, vitamin D		1 hr and 2 hr post prandial blood sugars (PC)
		Tissue transglutaminase (TTG) antibody		HbA1c

Imaging		
	Plain X-ray abdomen	
	Ultrasound abdomen	

ADRENAL GLAND

Mineralocorticoid excess

Basic tests			Additional tests		
	Sodium			Magnesium	
	Potassium			Saline infusion test	
	Bicarbonate				
	Creatinine				
	Renin				
	Aldosterone				
	Aldosterone/renin ratio				
Imaging					
	US and renal artery Doppler				
	CT scan/MRI				
	Adrenal venous sampling				

GLUCOCORTICOID EXCESS

Basic tests			Additional tests		
	Sodium, potassium, creatinine			Midnight cortisol	
	Fasting and postprandial blood sugar			Midnight ACTH	

Contd...

Contd...

	8 AM cortisol 24-hr urinary free cortisol (UFC) Urine cortisol/creatinine ratio		Low dose (1 mg) dexamethasone suppression test	8 AM Cortisol & ACTH, 24-hr urinary free cortisol
	Calcium, phosphorus, albumin, alkaline phosphatase and vitamin D		High dose (8 mg) dexamethasone suppression test	8 AM Cortisol & ACTH, 24-hr urinary free cortisol
Imaging				
	CT adrenals +/- CT thorax			
	PET scan			
	Bone density			
Androgen excess				
Basic tests	Suspected congenital adrenal hyperplasia (CAH)			
	Sodium, potassium			
	Cortisol (basal and post-Synacthen)			
	17 OH P (basal and post-Synacthen)			
	DHEAS (basal and post-Synacthen)			
	Suspected tumors			
	DHEAS, testosterone			
Imaging				
	CT scan/MRI			

PHEOCHROMOCYTOMA				
Basic tests			Additional tests	
	Serum catecholamines (or) serum metanephrines			Calcitonin
	24-hr urinary metanephrine and normetanephrine			Calcium, phosphorus, albumin, parathyroid hormone (PTH)

Contd...

Contd...

Imaging			
	Metaiodobenzylguanidine (MIBG) scan	Genetic analysis. Look for the following mutations	Rearranged during transfection (RET), von Hippel-Lindau (VHL), and succinate dehydrogenase (SDH) mutations.
	CT scan/MRI		

OVARY			
Basic tests		Additional tests	
	FSH		Inhibin
	LH		Anti-Müllerian hormone (AMH)
	Prolactin		GnRH stimulation test
	Estradiol		Karyotyping
Imaging			Cancer antigen (CA)-125
	Ultrasound and MRI pelvis		

TESTIS			
Basic tests		Additional tests	
	Testosterone		GnRH stimulation test
	SHBG		hCG stimulation test
	FSH		
	LH		
	Prolactin		
	Semen analysis		
Imaging			
	Ultrasound		

PITUITARY			
Basic tests		Hormone assays	
	PCV		Total T_4, Free T_4, TSH
	Blood sugars and HbA1c		Cortisol (8 AM)
	Sodium, potassium, creatinine		FSH, LH, prolactin (in dilution)
	Calcium, phosphorus		Testosterone (8 AM)
	Albumin		SHBG
	Lipid profile		HGH

Contd...

Contd...

			IGF-1
Imaging			
	MRI pituitary		

ACROMEGALY

Specific tests			Follow up: HGH (basal, 1 hr and 2-hr post-glucose), IGF-1, Prolactin
	HGH (basal)		
	IGF-1		
	Prolactin		
	HGH 1 hour & 2 hour post glucose (75 g)		
Other tests	ECG, ECHO		

CUSHING'S DISEASE

Specific tests			
	8 AM cortisol		
	8 AM ACTH		
	24 hour urinary cortisol		
	Midnight cortisol		
	Midnight ACTH		
	Low-dose dexasuppression test (1 mg)		8 AM cortisol, ACTH, 24-hr urinary cortisol
	High dose dexasuppression test (8 mg)		8 AM cortisol, ACTH, 24-hr urinary cortisol
Imaging			
	MRI pituitary with dynamic scan		On follow up: 1. Check 8 AM cortisol after stopping medication (Prednisolone for 48 hours or Hydrocortisone for 24 hours) 2. The Synacthen test is indicated for patients with borderline cortisol levels
	CT scan including chest and adrenals		
	PET scan		
	Inferior petrosal sinus sampling (IPSS)		

PROLACTINOMAS

Basic test		Other tests	
	Prolactin (in dilution)		Look for features MEN-1 • Calcium, phosphorus, PTH • Screen for pancreatic neuroendocrine tumors (PNET)

GONADOTROPH ADENOMAS			
Basic tests			
	FSH and LH		

NON-FUNCTIONING TUMORS			
Basic tests			
	Total T$_4$ and Free T$_4$		
	8 AM cortisol		
	Testosterone		

PREOPERATIVE ASSESSMENT	
Synacthen test	
	If the post-Synacthen cortisol >20 µg/dL, there is no need for perioperative steroid cover
	If the post-Synacthen cortisol <20 µg/dL, the patient will need hydrocortisone cover in the perioperative period.

POSTOPERATIVE HYPONATREMIA			
Basic tests			Diagnosis
	Serum sodium		
	Urine spot sodium		
	Serum osmolarity		
	Serum cortisol	<10 µg/dL	Hypocortisolemia
	N terminal pro-natriuretic peptide (NT-proBNP)	<125 pg/mL	Syndrome of antidiuretic hormone secretion (SIADH)
		>125 pg/mL	Cerebral salt wasting (CSW)

DIABETES INSIPIDUS			
Basic tests		Other tests	
	24-hr urine volume		Water deprivation test
	Serum sodium		
	Serum osmolarity		
	Urine osmolarity		
	Serum sodium after 12-hr water deprivation		
Imaging			
	MRI (Pituitary and hypothalamus)		
	Bone scan		
	PET scan		

CHAPTER 3

Endocrine Test Protocols

ASSESSMENT OF ANTERIOR PITUITARY FUNCTION

INSULIN TOLERANCE TEST[1]

Indications
- Assessment of adrenocorticotropic hormone (ACTH) and cortisol reserve
- Assessment of growth hormone reserve.

Contraindications
- Ischemic heart disease
- Epilepsy
- Severe hypothyroidism
- Serum cortisol < 3.6 µg/dL or < 100 nmol/L.

Prepubertal male and female children (with bone age >10 years) require testosterone/estrogen priming before the procedure
- *Male children require*: Testosterone enanthate 100 mg IM OD for 3 days.
- *Female children require*: Ethinyl estradiol 100 µg OD for 3 days.

Insulin dose required:
- *Normal pituitary function*: 0.15 U/kg
- *Hypopituitarism*: 0.1 U/kg
- *Acromegaly, Type 2 diabetes, Cushing's*: 0.2-0.3 U/kg.

Procedures
The patients should come on an empty stomach and should be resting prior to starting the procedure:
- An intravenous line is started and blood samples are collected for baseline (0') glucose, cortisol and growth hormone. The line is kept patent with an infusion of 0.9% normal saline 50 mL/hr.

- The patient is given an intravenous bolus of regular insulin as mentioned above. Glucometer reading is taken at 30 minutes and the insulin dose is repeated if the patient has not developed hypoglycemia by this time.
- Blood samples for glucose, cortisol and growth hormone are subsequently collected at 30, 60, 90 and 120 minutes intervals.
- Blood sugar levels are also constantly monitored at the bedside. The test should continue until the patient develops symptoms of hypoglycemia and the blood sugar levels drops to < 40 mg/dL (2.2 mmol/L).

NAME:
HOSPITAL NO:
DATE:

Minutes	Actual time	Medication	Glucometer readings	Blood tests	Symptoms
- 20					
- 5				Glucose, cortisol and growth hormone	
		Regular insulin 0.1 unit/kg IV			
0 min (when the patient develops symptoms and the blood sugar level is <40 mg/dL)				Glucose, cortisol and growth hormone	
+ 15				Glucose, cortisol and growth hormone	
+ 30				Glucose, cortisol and growth hormone	
+ 60				Glucose, cortisol and growth hormone	
+ 90				Glucose, cortisol and growth hormone	
+ 120				Glucose, cortisol and growth hormone	

Interpretations

- An adequate cortisol response is a rise >18 µg/dL (500 nmol/L).
- An adequate growth hormone response is a rise > 6 ng/mL (18 mIU/L) in adults and >12 ng/mL (36 mIU/L) in children.

GLUCAGON TEST[2]

Indications

This test is used to test the growth hormone and cortisol reserve in patient's in whom the insulin tolerance test (ITT) is contraindicated.

Contraindications

- Pheochromocytoma or insulinoma
- Severe hypothyroidism
- Serum cortisol < 100 nmol/L
- Starvation > 48 hours
- Chronic liver disease.

Glucagon dose
- *Adults*: 1 mg (1.5 mg if weight is >90 kg)
- *Children*: 15 µg/kg.

Procedures

- Patients come in after an over night fast.
- An indwelling cannula is inserted and blood samples are collected for basal glucose, growth hormone and cortisol.
- Patients are given inj. glucagon IM (as mentioned).
- Subsequent blood samples for growth hormone and cortisol are collected at 90, 120, 150 and 180 minutes.

NAME: HOSPITAL NO: DATE:					
Minutes	Actual time	Medication	Glucometer readings	Blood tests	Symptoms
- 20					
- 5				Glucose, cortisol and growth hormone	
		Inj. glucagon 1 mg IM			
+ 90				Glucose, cortisol and growth hormone	

Contd...

Contd...

Minutes	Actual time	Medication	Glucometer readings	Blood tests	Symptoms
+ 120				Glucose, cortisol and growth hormone	
+ 150				Glucose, cortisol and growth hormone	
+ 180				Glucose, cortisol and growth hormone	

Interpretations
- An adequate cortisol response is a rise >18 µg/dL (500 mol/L).
- An adequate Growth hormone response is a rise >6 ng/mL (18 mIU/L) in adults and >12 ng/mL (36 mIU/L) in children.

CLONIDINE TEST[3]

Indication
This test is used to test the growth hormone reserve when insulin tolerance test is contraindicated.

Precaution
The patients should continue to lie down for 2 hours after completing the test or until the blood pressure readings are satisfactory.

Clonidine dose: 0.15 mg/m².

Procedures
- Patients come in after fasting from midnight
- An indwelling cannula is inserted and a blood sample is collected for basal growth hormone
- The patient is given clonidine orally as mentioned, and the blood pressure is monitored every 30 minutes during the procedure
- Subsequent blood samples for growth hormone are collected at 30, 45, 60, 90, 120 and 150 minutes.

Interpretation
An adequate growth hormone response is a rise >10 ng/mL (30 mIU/L).

GONADOTROPIN RELEASING HORMONE ANALOG TEST[4-6]

Indications

- To assess the pituitary gonadotropin response in disorders of puberty or gonadal function
- To distinguish central precocious puberty (CPP) from peripheral precocious puberty (PPP).

Gonadotropin releasing hormone (GnRH) analog dose: 100 µg (triptorelin or decapeptyl); 20 µg/kg (leuprolide).

Procedures

- An indwelling cannula is inserted and blood samples are collected for baseline luteinizing hormone (LH), follicle-stimulating hormone (FSH), Estradiol (females) and testosterone (males)
- Patients are then given triptorelin 100 µg subcutaneously or Leuprolide 20 µg/kg subcutaneously (maximum dose 500 µg)
- Subsequently blood samples for LH, FSH, estradiol (in girls) and testosterone (in boys) are collected once at 60 minutes and again after 24 hours.

Interpretations

- The normal basal reference values in prepubertal children are LH < 0.2 IU/L and FSH < 2 IU/L.
- Normal prepubertal children will not respond to GnRH stimulation unlike children with underlying precocious puberty.
- The diagnosis of central precocious puberty is confirmed if at LH > 5 mIU/mL and FSH > 2 mIU/mL at 60 minutes, and estradiol >10 pg/mL (in girls) and testosterone > 25 ng/dL (in boys) at 24 hours.

ACROMEGALY[7]

ORAL GLUCOSE TOLERANCE TEST

Indication

When there is a suspicion of acromegaly or gigantism.

Precaution

Normal plasma glucose and well-controlled diabetes.

Procedures

- The patient should remain fasting from midnight.

- An indwelling cannula is inserted and blood samples are collected for baseline growth hormone, IGF-1 and glucose
- The patient is administered 75 g of oral glucose in 300 mL of water.
- Subsequently blood samples for growth hormone and glucose are collected at 30, 60, 90 and 120 minutes.

NAME: HOSPITAL NO: DATE:					
Minutes	Actual time	Medication	Glucometer readings	Blood tests	Symptoms
- 20					
- 5				Glucose, growth hormone and IGF-1	
		75 g oral glucose			
+ 30				Glucose and growth hormone	
+ 60				Glucose and growth hormone	
+ 90				Glucose and growth hormone	
+ 120				Glucose and growth hormone	

Interpretation

In normal individuals growth hormone levels fall to undetectable levels (< 0.4 ng/mL) after the ingestion of glucose. Failure to suppress growth hormone or a paradoxical rise in growth hormone levels suggests underlying acromegaly.

ASSESSMENT OF THE GROWTH HORMONE STATUS AFTER SURGERY

THE DEFINITION OF CURE

A. Immediately after surgery:
1. Mean growth hormone on a 5 point day curve checked at 09:00 hr, 11:00 hr, 13:00 hr, 15:00 hr and 17:00 hr should be <1.7 ng/mL.
2. Growth hormone nadir <0.4 µg/L after oral glucose tolerance test (OGTT).

B. After 12 weeks:
Reassess the IGF-1 status.

CUSHING'S DISEASE[8]

Normally the highest ACTH and cortisol levels are reached in the morning between 6 AM and 8 AM, the lowest ACTH and cortisol levels occur around midnight. This pattern is lost in patients with Cushing's disease.

ESTABLISHING THE HYPERCORTISOLEMIC STATE

24-HOUR URINARY FREE CORTISOL

Normal 24-hour urinary cortisol levels can range up to 55 µg. Levels >3 times the upper limit are diagnostic of Cushing's syndrome.

NIGHT-TIME SALIVARY CORTISOL

The diagnosis of Cushing's syndrome is confirmed if the salivary cortisol level at bedtime is >1 µg/dL and the level at midnight is >0.27 µg/dL.

MIDNIGHT CORTISOL AND ACTH

If the patient is sleeping, midnight serum cortisol >1.8 µg/dL confirms the diagnosis of Cushing's syndrome. If the patient is awake, a level >7.5 µg/dL confirms the diagnosis of Cushing's syndrome.

If the ACTH level is >7.5 pg/mL at the same time, it points towards an underlying pituitary tumor (ACTH-dependent Cushing's disease), very rarely it could be an ectopic ACTH secreting tumor.

If the ACTH level is <7.5 pg/mL, it points toward an underlying adrenal lesion either a unilateral adrenal adenoma or nodular adrenal hyperplasia which is usually bilateral (ACTH-independent Cushing's syndrome).

OVERNIGHT DEXAMETHASONE SUPPRESSION TEST

Indication
Initial screening test for patients with Cushing's syndrome.

Contraindications
- Pregnancy
- Patients on Hormone replacement therapy (HRT) or oral contraceptives (should stop treatment for 6 weeks)
- Patients on anticonvulsants
- Patients on rifampicin.

Procedures

- The patient takes 1 mg of dexamethasone at 23:00 hour.
- Serum cortisol is collected at 09:00 hour on the following day.

Interpretation

Failure to suppress cortisol to <1.8 µg/dL (50 nmol/L) confirms the diagnosis of endogenous Cushing's.

LOW-DOSE DEXAMETHASONE SUPPRESSION TEST

Indications

- Screening test for Cushing's syndrome when the overnight dexamethasone suppression test is positive.
- To differentiate women with excess testosterone due to polycystic ovary syndrome (PCOS) and congenital adrenal hyperplasia (CAH—partial hydroxylase deficiency) from those with androgen secreting tumors.

Contraindications

- Pregnancy
- Patients on HRT or oral contraceptives (should stop treatment for 6 weeks)
- Patients on anticonvulsants
- Patients on rifampicin.

Procedures

- On the first day blood samples are collected for baseline cortisol and ACTH at 09:00 hours.
- After this the patient takes tablet dexamethasone 0.5 mg at 6 hourly intervals for 48 hours.
- 6 hours after the last dose of dexamethasone, the second set of blood samples (at 48 hours) are collected for cortisol and ACTH (Similarly blood samples are collected for testosterone and DHEAS for patients being evaluated for androgen excess).

Interpretations

Failure to suppress serum cortisol levels to <1.8 µg/dL (50 nmol/L) confirms the diagnosis of endogenous Cushing's.

Women with PCOS and partial hydroxylase deficiency show partial or complete suppression of testosterone, while those with underlying ovarian and adrenal androgen secreting tumors do not respond.

DEXA-CRH TEST[9]

Indication

To differentiate Cushing's syndrome from pseudo-Cushing's syndrome.

Procedures

- The patient is administered dexamethasone 0.5 mg 6 hourly for 48 hours
- Two hours after the last dose of dexamethasone the patient receives inj. CRH 1 µg/kg
- Blood samples for ACTH and cortisol are collected after 1 hour.

Interpretations

- Patients with pseudo-Cushing's syndrome will not respond to CRH.
- In patients with Cushing's syndrome the ACTH level will be > 27 pg/mL and the cortisol level will be > 1.4 µg/dL.

CRH STIMULATION TEST[10]

Indication

To identify patients with Cushing's disease.

Procedures

- The patient should come in after an overnight fast
- An indwelling cannula is inserted and blood samples are collected for baseline ACTH and Cortisol at 8:30 AM
- The patient receives ovine or human CRH 1 µg/kg intravenously
- Subsequently blood samples for ACTH and Cortisol are collected after 15, 30, 45, 60, 90 and 120 minutes
- While normal individuals show a 10–15% increase in ACTH and cortisol levels
- In patients with Cushing's disease, ACTH levels will increase >50% and cortisol levels will increase >20%.

INVESTIGATING THE CAUSE OF CUSHING'S SYNDROME

HIGH-DOSE DEXAMETHASONE SUPPRESSION TEST[11]

Indication

To identify patients with Cushing's disease.

Contraindications

- Pregnancy

- Patients on HRT or oral contraceptives (should stop treatment for 6 weeks)
- Patients on anticonvulsants
- Patients on Rifampicin.

Procedures
- On the first day blood samples are collected for baseline cortisol and ACTH at 09:00 hour
- After this the patient takes tablet dexamethasone 2 mg 6 hourly for 48 hours
- 6 hours after the last dose of dexamethasone, the second set of blood samples are collected for cortisol and ACTH at 09:00 hour.

Interpretations
If serum cortisol levels are suppressed below 50% it confirms the diagnosis of Cushing's disease. Those with underlying adrenal and ectopic tumors will not respond to high dose dexamethasone.

INFERIOR PETROSAL SINUS SAMPLING (IPSS)[12]

Indication
To confirm the diagnosis of Cushing's disease and localize the tumor.

Procedures
- The patient is permitted only clear liquids after midnight on the day of the procedure.
- Each Petrosal sinus is catheterized separately using the femoral approach.
- Blood for ACTH is obtained simultaneously from each Petrosal sinus and from a peripheral site for comparison. At different time points (i) before CRH, (ii) 3–5 minutes after CRH, and (iii) 10 minutes after CRH [dose 1 µg/kg (maximum 100 µg IV)].

Interpretations
Cushing's disease is confirmed when the central to peripheral ACTH ratio is 2:1, and there is further increment to 3:1 after CRH stimulation.

ASSESSMENT OF REMISSION OF CUSHING'S DISEASE

DESMOPRESSIN TEST[13]

Indication
Assessment of patients who have had surgery for Cushing's disease.

Procedures

- The patient should come after an overnight fast
- An indwelling cannula is inserted and blood samples are collected for baseline ACTH and cortisol at 8:30 AM
- The patient is then administered 10 μg Desmopressin IV
- Subsequently blood samples for ACTH and cortisol are collected at 15, 30, 45, 60, 90 and 120 minutes.

Interpretation

A positive ACTH response indicates residual disease.

CORTISOL DAY CURVE[14]

Indication

To assess remission after trans-sphenoidal pituitary surgery for Cushing's disease.

Preparation

The last dose of hydrocortisone is taken at mid-day on the day before the test. Patients are advised to omit hydrocortisone on the day of the test.

Procedure

After inserting a cannula blood samples for serum cortisol are collected at 09:00, 12:00, 15:00 and 18:00 hours.

Interpretation

The mean serum cortisol should range between 5.4–10.9 μg/dL (150–300 nmol/L).

POSTERIOR PITUITARY

In a normal individual the plasma osmolality will range from 280 to 295 mOsmol/kg.

WATER DEPRIVATION TEST[15]

Do not proceed with the test if the patient's baseline plasma osmolality is >295 mOsmol/kg, serum sodium > 140 mmol/L and urine osmolality is <300 mOsmol/kg (hypotonic).

Preparations

- No tobacco or alcohol for 24 hours
- Stop DDAVP 24 hours prior to starting the test

- Patient can have a light breakfast (do not fast or limit fluids overnight)
- The test will continue from 8:30 hr to 20:30 hr, no fluids will be allowed until 16:30 hour.

Procedure

Stage 1 (8:00-16:30 hr)
- Insert an indwelling cannula and collect baseline sample for serum osmolality and serum sodium at 8:00 hour.
- Weight the patient at time '0' and calculate 97% of his body weight. Continue to monitor his weight at one hour intervals. The test should be discontinued if he loses more than 3% of his body weight.
- Urine is passed and discarded at time '0'. Subsequent urine samples are collected at one hour intervals and their volume is documented and the specimen is sent to the lab for measuring urine osmolality.
- Subsequent blood samples for serum osmolality and serum sodium are collected at 9:00, 12:00, 15:00 and 16:00 hour.

Stage 2 (16:30-20:30 hr)
- The patient is allowed to eat and drink freely.
- At 16:30 hour the patient receives aqueous vasopressin 5 units SC or Desmopressin 2 µg IM or 20 µg intranasally.
- Continue to measure hourly urine volume and urine osmolarity until the end of the procedure.

WATER DEPRIVATION TEST					
Time	Weight (kg)	Urine volume (mL)	Serum sodium	Serum osmolality (mOsmol/kg)	Urine osmolality (mOsmol/kg)
08:00					
09:00					
10:00					
11:00					
12:00					
13:00					
14:00					
15:00					
16:00					
If urine osmolality at 16:00 is <600 mOsmol/kg, the patient is given desmopressin 20 µg intranasally or 2 µg IM at 16:30					
DESMOPRESSIN TEST					
Time	Weight (kg)	Urine volume (mL)	Serum sodium	Serum osmolality (mOsmol/kg)	Urine osmolality (mOsmol/kg)
17:30					

Contd...

Contd...

Time	Weight (kg)	Urine volume (mL)	Serum sodium	Serum osmolality (mosmol/kg)	Urine osmolality (mosmol/kg)
18:30					
19:30					
20:30					

Interpretation

- *Normal response to dehydration*: Serum osmolality increases but is <300 mOsmal/kg. Urine osmolality increases >600 mOsmol/kg.
- *Partial DI*: In stage 1 serum osmolality increases but does not exceed 300 mOsmol/kg whereas urine remains dilute.
- *Complete DI*: Serum osmolality exceeds 300 mOsmol/kg while the urine remains dilute.

Response to Desmopressin

- *Central DI*: Urine concentration increases >150% of the highest earlier reading.
- *Nephrogenic DI*: No response to desmopressin.

POSTDEHYDRATION OSMOLALITY (MOSMOL/KG)		POST-DDAVP OSMOLALITY (MOSMOL/KG)	DIAGNOSIS
Plasma	Urine	Urine	
283–293	>750	>750	Normal
>293	<300	<300	Nephrogenic DI
>293	<300	>750	Central DI
<293	300–750	<750	Chronic polydipsia
<293	300–750	<750	Partial nephrogenic DI or Primary polydipsia
>293	300–750	>750	Partial central DI

MEDULLARY THYROID CARCINOMA

CALCIUM INFUSION TEST[16]

Preparation

The patient should come in after an overnight fast.

Procedures

- An intravenous cannula is inserted and a blood sample is collected for basal calcitonin
- The patient is then given calcium gluconate 0.2 mL/kg slow IV over 1 minute

- Subsequently blood samples are collected for calcitonin at 1, 2, 3, 5 and 10 minutes.

Interpretation
The normal range for calcitonin after calcium infusion is 100–200 ng/L.

PANCREAS

ORAL GLUCOSE TOLERANCE TEST FOR ASSESSMENT OF DIABETIC STATUS

Preparations
- Normal carbohydrate diet (>150 g/day) for 3 days
- The patient must fast for 10–14 hours before the test.

Procedure
- *0 min*: 1–2 mL blood is collected for plasma glucose.
    - The patient then drinks a solution containing 75 g glucose
- *120 min*: Second blood sample is collected for plasma glucose.

Interpretation

	Plasma glucose (mg/dL)	
	0 min	120 min
Nondiabetic	< 100	< 140
Prediabetes	100–125	140–200
Diabetes	>126	>200

48 OR 72 HOUR FAST[17]

Indications
To demonstrate fasting hypoglycemia and confirm the diagnosis of insulinoma.

Preparation
Explain the details of the test procedure and obtain the patient's consent.

Procedures
- An intravenous cannula is inserted and the patient commences the fast. They are allowed to drink water
- Blood glucose should be monitored at regular intervals (4-6 hrs) and whenever the patient has symptoms of hypoglycemia. When the blood

glucose falls below 3.0 mmol/L blood glucose should be monitored more frequently.
- When the blood glucose level reaches 40 mg/dL (2.2 mmol/L) and the patient develops symptoms of hypoglycemia collect blood samples for Insulin, C-peptide and sulfonylurea screening.
- If the patient does not develop hypoglycemia during the test period (72 hrs), ask him to exercise for 15–30 minutes and then collect the final samples for glucose, insulin, C-peptide and sulphonylurea screening.

NAME:			
HOSPITAL NO:			
Date	Time	Glucometer readings	Symptoms

When the blood glucose reaches 2.2 mmol/L or the patient develops symptoms of hypoglycemia, collect blood samples for insulin, C-peptide and sulfonylurea screening

Interpretations
- *Normal response*: Insulin 3–6 mU/L; C-peptide 300 ng/mL.
- *Insulinoma*: Insulin >6 mU/L; C-peptide >900 ng/mL.

ADRENAL GLAND

SHORT SYNACTHEN TEST[18]

Indications
- To detect the adrenal reserve in both primary and secondary hypoadrenalism.
- Confirm the diagnosis of CAH.

Preparations
- The patient should stop hydrocortisone the night before the test and should also skip his usual morning dose.
- HRT and estrogen therapy should be discontinued 6 weeks before the test.

Procedures

- An indwelling cannula is inserted and blood samples are collected for baseline ACTH and cortisol at 09:00 hour. For patients with suspected congenital adrenal hyperplasia (CAH), samples are also collected for baseline 17-OH progesterone (17-OHP) and DHEAS.
- The patient is given 250 µg of synacthen IM or IV.
- Subsequently, repeat blood samples for cortisol and 17-OH progesterone are collected at 30 and 60 minutes (09:30 and 10:00 hr).

NAME: HOSPITAL NO: DATE:				FOR PATIENTS WITH SUSPECTED CAH
Minutes	Actual time	Medication	Blood test	
-20				
-5			Cortisol	17 OHP and DHEAS
-0		Synacthen 250 µg IM		
+30			Cortisol	
+60			Cortisol	17 OHP and DHEAS

Interpretations

- *Normal response*: Stimulated plasma cortisol >20 µg/dL (or) an incremental rise of at least 6 µg/dL
- *Primary adrenal insufficiency*: Impaired cortisol response and ACTH >200 pg/mL
- *Secondary adrenal insufficiency*: ACTH < 10 pg/mL and varied cortisol response
- In patients with 21 hydroxylase deficiency, the response will vary depending whether they carry a homozygous or heterozygous mutation.

ACTON PROLONGATUM MAY BE USED INSTEAD OF SYNACTHEN[19]

Acton prolongatum is synthetic corticotrophin (of porcine sequence).

Procedures

- An indwelling cannula is inserted and blood samples are collected for baseline ACTH and cortisol
- Injection acton prolongatum is available as 60 units/mL
- Using a 40 IU/mL insulin syringe load up to the level 16 and inject 25 units intramuscularly
- The second blood sample is collected after 60 minutes for estimation of cortisol.

Interpretation

1 hour post-injection cortisol levels <18 µg/dL (500 nmol/L) indicates adrenal insufficiency.

SALINE INFUSION TEST[20]

Indication

To confirm primary hyperaldosteronism.

Contraindications

- Cardiac failure
- Uncontrolled hypertension
- Renal insufficiency
- Severe hypokalemia
- Cardiac arrhythmias.

Preparations

- Stop spironolactone and eplerenone 6 weeks prior to the test.
- Stop diuretics, beta blockers, calcium channel antagonists, ACE inhibitors and ARBs 2 weeks prior to the test.
- Ensure plasma potassium is >4 mmol/L.
- Patients stay recumbent for at least 1 hour prior to starting the test.

Procedures

- An indwelling cannula is inserted and blood samples are collected for baseline urea, electrolytes, aldosterone and renin
- Starting at 09:00 hr, infuse 2 L of 0.9% saline over 4 hours
- Monitor heart rate, blood pressure and oxygen saturation throughout the procedure
- After finishing the infusion (13:00 hr) repeated blood samples are collected for electrolytes, aldosterone and renin.

Interpretations

- *Normal response*: Post-infusion aldosterone levels < 5 pg/mL
- *Primary hyperaldosteronism*: Post-infusion aldosterone levels > 10 pg/mL.

TESTIS

HUMAN CHORIONIC GONADOTROPIN STIMULATION TEST[21]

Indications

- To determine Leydig cell responsiveness in primary hypogonadism.
- To identify the presence or absence of testicular tissue in cryptorchidism.

hCG Dose
- *Under 2 years*: Single intramuscular injection 1500 IU
- *Above 2 years*: Single intramuscular injection 5000 IU.

Procedures
- Collect pre-hCG blood sample for testosterone (T) and dihydrotestosterone (DHT)
- Administer hCG mixed with 1% lignocaine
- Post-hCG blood samples are collected between 72–96 hours for T and DHT.

	Testosterone (T)	Dihydrotestosterone (DHT)	T/DHT ratio following hCG
Normal adult males	8–27 nmol/L	<2–9 nmol/L	<12
Normal children (6 months–puberty)	<0.9 nmol/L	<0.1 nmol/L	<12
5-alpha reductase deficiency (6 months–puberty)	<0.5 nmol/L		>12

Interpretations
- *Normal response*: Stimulated testosterone >3-fold above baseline. Inadequate response suggests Leydig cell failure.
- Normal (mean) T/DHT ratio = 10, range (2–20)
- Poor DHT response and elevated post-hCG T/DHT ratio suggests underlying 5-alpha reductase deficiency.

CARCINOID TUMORS

- *Chromogranin A (CgA)*: Normal range in blood is <36.4 ng/mL. Chromogranin A is useful in the evaluation of patients with suspected carcinoid tumors, pancreatic neuroendocrine tumors (PNETs) and pheochromocytomas.
- 5-Hydroxyindoleacetic acid (5-HIAA)—the normal range in a 24-hour urine collection is <6 mg
- During the 24-hour urine collection for 5-HIAA the following food items and drugs should be avoided:
  - *Fruits and nuts*: Including bananas, tomatoes, pineapples, avocados, plums and walnuts.
  - *Drugs*: Including paracetamol, heparin, isoniazid, monoamine oxidase inhibitors, methyldopa, phenothiazines and tricyclic antidepressants.

REFERENCES

1. Greenwood FC, Landon J, Stamp TC. The plasma sugar, free fatty acid, cortisol, and growth hormone response to insulin. I. In control subjects. J Clin Invest. 1966;45(4):429-36.
2. Rao RH, Spathis GS. Intramuscular glucagon as a provocative stimulus for the assessment of pituitary function: Growth hormone and cortisol responses. Metabolism. 1987;36(7):658-63.
3. Rahim A, Toogood AA, Shalet SM. The assessment of growth hormone status in normal young adult males using a variety of provocative agents. Clin Endocrinol (Oxf). 1996;45(5):557-62.
4. Dash RJ, Sialy R, Rao NS. LH and FSH responses to GnRH in health and disease. J Steroid Biochem. 1985;23(5B):823-6.
5. Bajpai A. Precocious puberty. In: Desai MP, Bhatia V, Menon PSN (Eds). Pediatric Endocrine. Disorders, 1st edn. New Delhi: Orient Longman; 2001. pp. 217-41.
6. Freire AV, Escobar ME, Gryngarten ME, et al. High diagnostic accuracy of subcutaneous Triptorelin test compared with GnRH test for diagnosing central precocious puberty in girls. Clin Endocrinol. 2013;78(3):398-404.
7. American Association of Clinical Endocrinologists Medical Guidelines for Clinical Practice for the Diagnosis and Treatment of Acromegaly-2011 Update- Endocrine Practice - Volume 17, Supplement 4 / July-August 2011 - American Association of Clinical Endocrinologists. Available from: http://aace.metapress.com/content/5h1427154k550851/
8. Nieman LK, Biller BMK, Findling JW, et al. The diagnosis of Cushing's syndrome: an endocrine society clinical practice guideline. J Clin Endocrinol Metab. 2008;93(5):1526-40.
9. The Dexamethasone-Suppressed Corticotrophin-Releasing Hormone Stimulation Test Differentiates Mild Cushing's Disease from Normal Physiology. Available from: http://press.endocrine.org/doi/pdf/10.1210/jcem.83.2.4568
10. Müller OA, Stalla GK, von Werder K. Corticotrophin releasing factor: a new tool for the differential diagnosis of Cushing's syndrome. J Clin Endocrinol Metab. 1983;57(1):227-9.
11. Tyrrell JB, Findling JW, Aron DC, et al. An overnight high-dose dexamethasone suppression test for rapid differential diagnosis of Cushing's syndrome. Ann Intern Med. 1986;104(2):180-6.
12. Bilateral Inferior Petrosal Sinus Sampling in Cushing's syndrome. Neuroendocrine Clinical Center & Pituitary Tumor Center at MGH/Harvard. Available from: http://pituitary.mgh.harvard.edu/E-F-932.HTM
13. Moro M, Putignano P, Losa M, et al. The desmopressin test in the differential diagnosis between Cushing's disease and pseudo-Cushing states. J Clin Endocrinol Metab. 2000;85(10):3569-74.
14. Trainer PJ, Eastment C, Grossman AB, et al. The relationship between cortisol production rate and serial serum Cortisol estimation in patients on medical therapy for Cushing's syndrome. Clin Endocrinol (Oxf). 1993;39(4):441-3.
15. Thompson CJ. Polyuric states in man. Baillières Clin Endocrinol Metab. 1989;3(2):473-97.
16. Parthemore JG, Bronzert D, Roberts G, et al. A short calcium infusion in the diagnosis of medullary thyroid carcinoma. J Clin Endocrinol Metab. 1974;39(1):108-11.

17. Bon AC, Benhadi N, Endert E, et al. Evaluation of Endocrine Tests. D: the prolonged fasting test for Insulinoma. Neth J Med. 2009;67(7):274-8.
18. Clark PM, Neylon I, Raggatt PR, et al. Defining the normal cortisol response to the short Synacthen test: implications for the investigation of hypothalamic-pituitary disorders. Clin Endocrinol (Oxf). 1998;49(3):287-92.
19. Gundgurthi A, Garg MK, Dutta MK, et al. Intramuscular ACTH stimulation test for assessment of adrenal function. J Assoc Physicians India. 2013;61(320):e324.
20. Mulatero P, Milan A, Fallo F, et al. Comparison of confirmatory tests for the diagnosis of primary aldosteronism. J Clin Endocrinol Metab. 2006;91(7):2618-23.
21. Davenport M, Brain C, Vandenberg C, et al. The use of the hCG stimulation test in the endocrine evaluation of cryptorchidism. Br J Urol. 1995;76(6):790-4.

CHAPTER 4

Treatment Protocols

HYPONATREMIA[1]

Classification

- Symptomatic or asymptomatic
- Acute (<48 hr) or chronic (>48 hr)
- Mild (130-134 mmol/L); moderate (125-129 mmol/L); severe < 125 mmol/L.

	Serum sodium (mmol/L)	Plasma osmolality (mOsmol/kg)	Cause
Hypotonic	<135	Low (<280)	SIADH, heart failure, cirrhosis
Isotonic	<135	Normal (280–295)	Hyperglycemia, psuedohyponatremia
Hypertonic	<135	High (>295)	Severe hyperglycemia with dehydration

Calculation

Total body water	
Children	0.6 x weight
Women	0.5 x weight
Men	0.6 x weight
Elderly women	0.45 x weight
Elderly men	0.5 x weight

Normal sodium = 140 mmol/L
Sodium deficit = (Desired sodium − Patient's sodium)
When half correction is planned = (Desired sodium − Patient's sodium)/2
Total body deficit of sodium (TBD) = Sodium deficit × (Weight in kgs × 0.6)
Most physicians replace the Sodium deficit at the rate of 0.5 mEq/hr.
Rate of replacement (hr) = Sodium deficit /0.5

SODIUM CONTENT OF INTRAVENOUS FLUIDS		
Fluid	Sodium content (mEq/L)	Sodium concentration (mEq/mL)
Ringer lactate	130	0.13
0.9% NaCl	154	0.154
3% NaCl	513	0.513

Fluid replacement per hour
= Total body deficit/sodium concentration per mL/ Rate of replacement
(Or)
= Sodium requirement (mmol) × 1000/infusate sodium (mmol/L) × time (hr).

Treatment

- The increase in serum sodium should not exceed 8 mmol/L in 24 hours, as rapid correction can lead to central pontine myelinolysis.
- *Patients with euvolemic, asymptomatic hyponatremia*: Restrict free water intake to 1 L per day.
- Patients with acute severe hyponatremia are given a bolus of 100 mL hypertonic saline over 10-15 minutes; this is followed by a slow infusion at the rate of 15-30 mL/hr.
- Patients with chronic severe hyponatremia are given a bolus of 50 mL hypertonic saline; this is followed by a slow infusion at the rate of 15-30 mL/hr. Some authors add desmopressin 1-2 µg SC/ IV 8 hourly for 28-48 hours.

HYPERNATREMIA[2]

Classification

- Acute (<48 hr)
- Chronic (>48 hr).

Calculation

Desired sodium = 140 mmol/L
Insensible water loss = 500-1500 mL/day
The maximum rate at which serum sodium should be lowered is 10-12 mmol/L per day.

> **Adrogue formula**
> Change in serum sodium = (Infusate sodium + Infusate potassium) − Serum sodium / (Total body water + 1)

Total water deficit (L) = Total body water × (1− Desired sodium/ serum sodium)

Desired water replacement on the first day
= Total water deficit × 10/(Serum sodium−Desired sodium)
Hourly infusion rate = Desired water replacement on the first day/24
All calculations should also account for the insensible water loss.

Treatment

- Acute hypernatremia— 5% dextrose at the rate of 3-6 mL/kg/hr
- Chronic hypernatremia—5% dextrose at the rate of 1.35 mL/kg/hr
- Once the serum sodium level reaches 145 mmol/L the infusion rate is reduced to 1 mL/kg/hr until the serum sodium level normalizes.
- Patients with central diabetes insipidus will require desmopressin.

HYPOKALEMIA[3]

Classification

- Mild (3-3.4 mmol/L)
- Moderate (2.5-2.9 mmol/L)
- Severe <2.5 mmol/L (or) with symptoms.

Treatment

- *Mild to moderate hypokalemia*:
    - 10-20 mmol of potassium chloride given 2-4 times a day.
- Severe hypokalemia warrants intravenous replacement, 40 mmol potassium chloride in 1L of 0.9% NaCl given twice or thrice daily.
    - Standard infusion rate 10 mmol/hr.
    - Maximum infusion rate 20 mmol/hr.
- *If the patient has hypomagnesemia in addition*: First give a bolus of 4 mL (8 mmol) of 50% $MgSO_4$ diluted in 10 mL 0.9% NaCl over 20 minutes and then start the potassium infusion. Continue magnesium infusion as per protocol.

HYPERKALEMIA[4]

Classification

- Mild (5.5-6 mmol/L)
- Moderate (6.1-7 mmol/L)
- Severe (>7 mmol/L)
- Asymptomatic/Symptomatic
- Acute/Chronic.

Treatment

- 10 mL of 10% calcium gluconate infused over 5 minutes, if necessary repeat at 5 and 10 minutes until ECG improves.

- 5–10 units soluble insulin with 50 mL of 50% dextrose (25 g glucose) over 5–10 minutes.
- Salbutamol 10–20 mg in 4 mL of 0.9% NaCl given as nebulization over 10 minutes.
- Calcium resonium or kayexalate (sodium polystyrene sulfonate) 15 g TID (with lactulose).
- If sodium bicarbonate is required, 50–100 mL of 8.4% sodium bicarbonate is given over 1 hour.

HYPOCALCEMIA[5]

Classification

- Mild 7.6–8.5 mg/dL (or) asymptomatic
- Severe <7.6 mg/dL (or) symptomatic.

Note:
- 10 mL of calcium gluconate (10%) contains 90 mg of elemental calcium.
- Tablets like Sandocal with 1250 mg of calcium carbonate contain 500 mg of elemental calcium.

Mild Hypocalcemia

- Tablet Sandocal—2 tablets BD.
- Following thyroidectomy if the serum calcium remains <8.4 mg/dL (<2.1 mmol/L)
  - Increase Sandocal to 2 tablets TID
  - If the patient remains hypocalcemic beyond 48 hours, commence 1,25 Vitamin D3 0.5–1 µg/day.
- If there is associated hypomagnesemia treat with 6 g $MgSO_4$ in 500 mL normal saline over 24 hours.

Severe Hypocalcemia

- 10–20 mL of calcium gluconate in 50–100 mL of 5% Dextrose over 10 minutes. This can be repeated until the patient is asymptomatic. Subsequently commence the patient on calcium infusion—dilute 100 mL of calcium gluconate (5 vials) in 500 mL of 0.9% NaCl and infuse at a rate of 50–100 mL/hr.
- Start 1,25 Vitamin D3 0.5–1 µg/day.
- Correct associated hypomagnesemia.

HYPERCALCEMIA[6]

Classification

- Mild <12 mg/dL
- Moderate 12–14 mg/dL
- Severe >14 mg/dL
- Asymptomatic/symptomatic.

Treatment

- Isotonic saline infused at a rate of 200–300 mL/hr in order to maintain urine output around 100–150 mL/hr.
- Salmon calcitonin 4 IU/kg repeated every 6–12 hours.
- Zoledronic Acid 4 mg IV over 15 minutes (or) pamidronic acid 60–90 mg over 2 hours.
- Patients with underlying sarcoidosis and lymphoma require prednisone 20–40 mg per day.

HYPOMAGNESEMIA[7]

Definition

Magnesium < 1.7 mg/dL.

Grading

Grade	1	2	3	4	5
Serum magnesium (mg/dL)	1.7–1.2	1.2–1	1–0.7	<0.7	Death

Treatment

- *Grade 1*: No treatment required
- *Grade 2*: 5 g $MgSO_4$ (20 mmol) in 500 mL normal saline over 6–8 hours. Oral magnesium supplements (Maalox) can be tried.
- *Grade 3 and 4*: 5 g $MgSO_4$ in 1 L normal saline over 8–10 hours. Repeat over the next 3–5 days until serum magnesium levels normalize (Reduce dose to 2.5 g $MgSO_4$ (10 mmol) for patients with renal impairment).

If hypocalcemic, correct magnesium until calcium comes within the normal range.

If hypokalemia, replace 40 mmol KCl and 1.25 g $MgSO_4$ (5 mmol) in 500 mL normal saline over 6 hours and repeat up to 24 hours until serum potassium levels improve.

ADRENAL INSUFFICIENCY[8]

Hydrocortisone replacement during stress and illness should not exceed 200 mg/day.

Surgical stress	Glucocorticoid dose
Minor	Hydrocortisone 25 mg IV at the start of the procedure, following the procedure continue the usual replacement dose
Moderate	Hydrocortisone 25 mg Q8H IV for 24 hr, subsequently taper the dose over the next 48 hr
Severe	Hydrocortisone 50 mg Q8H IV for 24 hours, subsequently taper the dose over the next 48–72 hr

REFERENCES

1. Spasovski G, Vanholder R, Allolio B, et al. Clinical practice guideline on diagnosis and treatment of hyponatremia. Eur J Endocrinol Eur Fed Endocr Soc. 2014;170(3):G1-47.
2. Adrogué HJ, Madias NE. Hypernatremia. N Engl J Med. 2000;342(20):1493-9.
3. Cohn JN, Kowey PR, Whelton PK, et al. New guidelines for potassium replacement in clinical practice: a contemporary review by the National Council on Potassium in Clinical Practice. Arch Intern Med. 2000;160(16):2429-36.
4. Elliott MJ, Ronksley PE, Clase CM, et al. Management of patients with acute hyperkalemia. Can Med Assoc J. 2010;182(15):1631-5.
5. Cooper MS, Gittoes NJL. Diagnosis and management of hypocalcaemia. Available from: http://www.ncbi.nlm.nih.gov/pmc/articles/PMC2413335/
6. AcuteHypercalcaemia.pdf. (Feb 2013) Available from: http://www.endocrinology.org/policy/docs/13-02_EmergencyGuidance-AcuteHypercalcaemia.
7. Martin KJ, González EA, Slatopolsky E. Clinical Consequences and Management of Hypomagnesaemia. Available from: http://jasn.asnjournals.org/content/20/11/2291.abstract
8. Arlt W. The approach to the adult with newly diagnosed adrenal insufficiency. J Clin Endocrinol Metab. 2009;94(4):1059-67.

CHAPTER 5

Endocrine Emergencies

THYROID STORM

Thyroid storm is a hypermetabolic state due to the excess release of thyroid hormones. It is a life-threatening condition precipitated by:
- Infection
- Trauma
- Surgery
- Noncompliance with medication
- Radioiodine therapy
- Diabetic ketoacidosis
- Toxemia of pregnancy
- Parturition

The diagnosis is based on clinical criteria defined by the Burch–Wartofsky score

Burch–Wartofsky score:

	Scoring points
Thermoregulatory dysfunction	
Temperature (°F)	
99–99.9	5
100–100.9	10
101–101.9	15
102–102.9	20
103–103.9	25
≥104	30
Cardiovascular dysfunction	
Tachycardia (beats/min)	
90–109	5
110–119	10
120–129	15
≥140	25

Contd...

Contd...

Congestive heart failure	
Absent	0
Mild (pedal edema)	5
Moderate (bibasilar rales)	10
Severe (pulmonary edema)	15
Gastrointestinal and hepatic dysfunction	
Absent	0
Moderate (diarrhea, abdominal pain, nausea/vomiting)	10
Severe (unexplained jaundice)	20
Central nervous system disturbance	
Absent	0
Mild (agitation)	10
Moderate (delirium, psychosis, extreme lethargy)	20
Severe (seizures, coma)	30
Precipitating event	
Absent	0
Present	10
Criteria	
Total score	
>45	Thyroid storm
25–44	Impending thyroid storm
< 25	Storm unlikely
Evaluation	
Thyroid profile	
CBC, LFT, electrolytes, urea, creatinine	
Other tests based on the clinical indication	
Treatment	
Beta blockers	• Propranolol 60–80 mg 4–6 hourly PO (or) • Esmolol 250–500 µg/kg (IV) bolus followed by an infusion at the rate of 50–100 µg/kg/hour • If beta blockers are contraindicated use diltiazem 60–90 mg 6–8 hourly PO, for control of heart rate
Propylthiouracil (or) Carbimazole	• Propylthiouracil 200 mg 4 hourly PO (or) • Carbimazole 20 mg 4–6 hourly PO

Contd...

Contd...

Oral iodine (or) Iodinated radio contrast agents	• Oral iodine: Lugol's iodine (10 drops) 1 mL TID x 7 days. Note: Lugol's iodine should always be commenced 1 hr after the 1st dose of propylthiouracil/carbimazole. (or) • Iodinated radio contrast agents: Ipodate or Iopanoic acid 500–1000 mg once daily PO.
Hydrocortisone	100 mg Q8H IV
Treatment of the underlying cause and supportive measures	

MYXEDEMA COMA

Myxedema coma is defined as severe hypothyroidism leading to altered sensorium. The hallmarks of myxedema coma include:
- Hypothermia
- Bradycardia
- Hypotension
- Hyponatremia
- Hypoglycemia (less common)
- Hypoventilation (less common)

Precipitating factors	*Important clues*
• Exposure to cold • Infection • Trauma • CNS depressant drugs and anesthetics • Myocardial infarction • Stroke	• Presence of a thyroidectomy scar • History of hypothyroidism • Prior radio iodine treatment
Evaluation	
• Thyroid profile • CBC • Blood glucose • Serum electrolytes • Creatinine	Other tests as indicated • Arterial blood gas • Septic screen • ECG
Treatment	

Thyroxine (oral /IV)
- Thyroxine 500 μg stat (PO or via NG tube), followed by 150 μg OD

  (or)
- IV Thyroxine 200–400 μg bolus followed by 50–100 μg OD.

  (or)
- Cytomel (T3) 5–20 μg stat (PO or via NG tube), followed by 2.5–10 μg Q8H.

Additional treatment
- Hydrocortisone 100 mg IV Q8H
- Broad spectrum antibiotic cover
- Treatment of severe hyponatremia (<120 mmol/L)
- Correction of hypoglycemia
- Treatment of hypotension
- Passive rewarming

HYPERCALCEMIA

Investigations (done prior to therapeutic intervention)

- Bone profile
- Parathyroid hormone
- Vitamin D
- Serum electrolytes
- Creatinine
- ECG

Classification

- Symptomatic/asymptomatic
- Acute/chronic
- Mild/moderate/severe

Category	Symptoms	Treatment
• *Mild*: Total calcium 10.5–11.9 mg/dL (Ionized calcium 1.4–2 mmol/L)	These patients are usually asymptomatic	• No intervention is required • Patients are asked to increase their fluid intake and come for follow-up in the outpatient clinic
• *Moderate*: Total calcium 12–13.9 mg/dL (Ionized calcium 2–2.5 mmol/L)	• These patients may or may not be symptomatic • Symptomatic patients complain of constipation, fatigue, malaise and depression	• Treatment is based on the clinical judgment • Those who need hospitalization are treated with intravenous fluids and IV Pamidronate

• *Severe*: Total calcium 14–16 mg/dL (Ionized calcium > 2.5 mmol/L)	These patients present with polyuria, polydipsia, dehydration, anorexia, nausea, muscle weakness and altered sensorium	They should be admitted and treated with Intravenous saline 4–6 L/day (Use with caution in elderly individuals and those with underlying cardiac and renal impairment. These patients will require close monitoring of their fluid status).
		• Bisphosphonates
		  – Pamidronate 60–90 mg diluted in 500 mL saline infused over 2 hr
		(or)
		  – Zolindronic acid 4 mg diluted in 100 mL saline infused over 15 minutes (Use caution in women in the reproductive age group and avoid in patients with underlying renal impairment).
		• Patients with underlying lymphoma and sarcoidosis require Prednisolone 20–40 mg/day.
		• Patients with refractory hypercalcemia will require dialysis

Endocrine Emergencies

HYPOCALCEMIA

Hypocalcemia is defined as serum calcium < 8.5 mg/dL or ionized calcium < 1.0 mmol/L. Depending on the duration and severity of hypocalcemia, these patients can develop:
- Tetany
- Paresthesias
- Seizures
- Neuropsychiatric manifestations

Causes	Investigations
• Hypoparathyroidism (post-surgery or idiopathic) • Vitamin D deficiency • Hypomagnesemia • Resistance to PTH action • Hyperphosphatemia • Acute pancreatitis • Hungry bone syndrome • Chemotherapy	• Bone profile • Parathyroid hormone (PTH) • Vitamin D_3 • Serum magnesium • ECG

Treatment

Patients with chronic asymptomatic hypocalcemia are treated as outpatients with oral calcium and vitamin D supplements.

Those with symptomatic hypocalcemia require prompt treatment with:
- Calcium gluconate 2 g (2 ampoules) IV over 10–20 minutes followed by calcium infusion 5 g (5 ampoules) diluted in 500 mL normal saline at the rate of 50 mL/hr (Monitor serum calcium 4 hourly and adjust the rate of infusion to maintain serum calcium levels between 8–8.8 mmol/L)
- Coexisting hypomagnesemia needs correction with magnesium sulfate 2 g IV bolus over 10–15 minutes, followed by an infusion at the rate of 1/hr
- These patients in addition should start on oral vitamin D and calcium supplements
- Patients with underlying hypoparathyroidism and renal impairment will need 1α-Calcidol or calcitriol 0.25–0.5 µg twice daily

ADRENAL INSUFFICIENCY

• Primary adrenal insufficiency (Addison's disease), is characterized by low cortisol and high ACTH • Secondary adrenal insufficiency which is due to hypothalamic or pituitary dysfunction is characterized by low cortisol and low ACTH	The clinical manifestations of this disorder can be acute or chronic. • The acute manifestation of adrenal insufficiency is with hyponatremia, hypotension and shock • The chronic manifestations include weakness, dizziness, anorexia, nausea, and vomiting and weight loss • Patients with primary adrenal insufficiency in addition will have increased pigmentation

Investigations

- Serum electrolytes, creatinine
- Cortisol (random), ACTH
- Ultrasound and CT scan of the adrenals—in patients with primary adrenal insufficiency

Contd...

Treatment
• During acute crises: Hydrocortisone 50 mg Q6H IV for 48–72 hr. • Maintenance dose: Hydrocortisone 10–12 mg/M^2 or 10-5-5 mg PO • Patients with primary adrenal insufficiency also require Fludrocortisone 100–200 µg OD

PHEOCHROMOCYTOMA

Patients with pheochromocytoma may present with:
• Headache
• Palpitation
• Sweating
• Anxiety
Hypertension may be sustained (50–60%) or paroxysmal (30%)
They can also present as:
• Cardiovascular emergencies with
   – Arrhythmias
   – Pulmonary edema
• Cerebrovascular accidents and seizures

Treatment of hypertensive crises

• Sodium nitroprusside infusion 0.25 µg/kg/min, the dose can be titrated up to 10 µg/kg/min. If sodium nitroprusside is not available start the patient on nitroglycerine infusion 5 µg/min and titrate the dose up to 100 µg/min to lower blood pressure to a safe level
• Magnesium sulfate 4 g over 5 minutes as an intravenous bolus, followed by an infusion at the rate of 1 g/hr
• Once the patient has stabilized add oral anti-hypertensive medication and gradually taper and stop the infusion
   – Phenoxybenzamine—starting with 10 mg twice daily, the dose can be increased by 10–20 mg every 2–3 days up to a maximum of 100 mg daily
   – Prazocin—starting with 1 mg twice daily, the dose can be increased up to 10 mg twice daily
   – Amlodipine 10–20 mg daily or Verapamil 180–540 mg daily

PITUITARY APOPLEXY
Is an acute emergency following infarction or hemorrhage into the pituitary gland. • The clinical syndrome could evolve over a few hours and can extend up to 3 days. • 50% of apoplectic events occur in patients not known to have pituitary tumors. • Untreated pituitary apoplexy is associated with high mortality.
Symptoms
• Severe headache • Nausea and vomiting • Vertigo • Ophthalmoplegia • Decreased visual acuity • Altered sensorium

Contd...

Contd...

Predisposing factors
• Head injury • Cabergoline or GnRH therapy • Anticoagulation • Major surgery • Pregnancy
Differential diagnosis
• Cerebral hemorrhage • Subarachnoid hemorrhage • Meningitis • Temporal arteritis • Diabetic 3rd nerve palsy • Hypertensive encephalopathy • Cavernous sinus thrombosis
Investigations
• Serum electrolytes • Creatinine • TFT • Cortisol (random) • Urgent MRI is the imaging modality of choice. However in the absence of a MRI scan, an urgent CT scan is advisable to exclude other diagnosis
Treatment
• Start IV Dexamethasone 4 mg Q8H while awaiting confirmation of diagnosis • Surgery is indicated for patients not responding to conservative management. This includes those with altered sensorium and deterioration in vision

DIABETES INSIPIDUS

Diabetes insipidus (DI) is characterized by the excretion of >3 L of dilute urine (<300 mOsm/kg) in 24 hr, accompanied by persistent thirst and hypernatremia (serum sodium >145 mmol/L)
Possible causes include:
- Central DI due to pituitary tumor/stalk lesions, surgery and head injury
- Nephrogenic DI can be due to renal disease or medication

Investigations

- Serum electrolytes
- Creatinine
- Serum osmolality
- Urine osmolality
- Serum cortisol
- MRI Pituitary
- PET scan (if indicated)

Treatment

Treatment will depend on the degree of hypernatremia and the presence or absence of symptoms.
- Patients who are asymptomatic and those with mild hypernatremia are started on DDAVP tablets 10–20 μg BD/TID or DDAVP nasal spray 100–400 μg BD/TID
- Patients who are symptomatic and those with serum sodium levels >150 mmol/L are treated with hypotonic saline infusion and DDAVP injections 1–2 μg SC BD
- The serum sodium level should not drop >10–12 mEq/L in 24 hours.

BIBLIOGRAPHY

1. AcuteHypercalcaemia.pdf. (Feb 2013) Available from: http://www.endocrinology.org/policy/docs/13-02_EmergencyGuidance-AcuteHypercalcaemia.
2. Arlt W. The approach to the adult with newly diagnosed adrenal insufficiency. J Clin Endocrinol Metab. 2009;94(4):1059-67.
3. Burch HB, Wartofsky L. Life-threatening thyrotoxicosis. Thyroid storm. Endocrinol Metab Clin North Am. 1993;22:263-77.
4. Carroll R, Matfin G. Endocrine and metabolic emergencies: thyroid storm. Ther Adv Endocrinol Metab. 2010;1(3):139-45.
5. Cooper MS, Gittoes NJL. Diagnosis and management of hypocalcaemia. Available from: http://www.ncbi.nlm.nih.gov/pmc/articles/PMC2413335/
6. Lenders JWM, Duh Q-Y, Eisenhofer G, et al. Pheochromocytoma and paraganglioma: an endocrine society clinical practice guideline. J Clin Endocrinol Metab. 2014;99(6):1915-42.
7. Mathew V, Misgar RA, Ghosh S, et al. Myxedema Coma: A New Look into an Old Crisis. J Thyroid Res; 2011. Available from: http://www.ncbi.nlm.nih.gov/pmc/articles/PMC3175396/
8. Nawar RN, Abdel Mannan D, Selman WR, et al. Pituitary tumor apoplexy: a review. J Intensive Care Med. 2008;23(2):75-90.
9. Rajaratnam S. Endocrine Emergencies—Textbook of Emergency Medicine. In: David, Brown, Nelson, Banerjee, Anantharaman, et al (Eds). Wolters Kluwer Health (Lippincott, Williams and Wilkins). 2012;1:336-45.
10. Verbalis JG. Diabetes Insipidus. Rev Endocr Metab Disord. 2003;4(2):177-85.

CHAPTER 6

Diabetes Protocols

DIAGNOSIS

DIABETES MELLITUS[1]	
HbA1c	≥6.5%
Fasting glucose	≥126 mg/dL
2-hr plasma glucose	≥200 mg/dL
Symptoms of hyperglycemia and a random plasma glucose	≥200 mg/dL

PREDIABETES	
Impaired fasting glucose (IFG)	
Fasting glucose	100–125 mg/dL
Impaired glucose tolerance (IGT)	
2-hr plasma glucose	140–199 mg/dL
HbA1c	
Prediabetic range	5.7–6.4%

ANTIBODY TITERS	
C-Peptide	1.1–5.0 ng/mL
Anti-GAD antibody	<5.0 U/mL
Anti-islet cell antibody	<7.5 U/mL
Zinc transporter 8 (ZnT8) islet antibody	10–500 U/mL

TARGETS FOR ADULTS WITH DIABETES[1]	
Blood sugar	
HbA1c	<7% for normal adults <6.5% for young healthy adults <8% for older adults with comorbidities
Preprandial capillary plasma glucose	80–130 mg/dL
Peak postprandial capillary plasma glucose	<180 mg/dL

Contd...

Contd...

Blood pressure	<140/90 mm Hg

Lipids	
LDL cholesterol	<100 mg/dL (<70 mg/dL in patients with underlying ischemic heart disease)
Triglycerides	<150 mg/dL
HDL cholesterol	Men >40 mg/dL
	Women >50 mg/dL

Targets for ICU patients
Blood glucose 140–180 mg/dL

CLASSIFICATION OF HYPOGLYCEMIA	
Level	Glycemic criteria
1.	≤70 mg/dL
2.	<54 mg/dL
3.	No specific glucose threshold
	The patient has severe cognitive impairment and needs external assistance for recovery

ORAL ANTIDIABETIC DRUGS[2]

Class	Medications
Sulfonylureas (SU)	Glibenclamide, glipizide gliclazide, glimiperide
Biguanides	Metformin
Meglitinides	Repaglinide, nateglinide
Alpha glucosidase inhibitors	Acarbose, voglibose
Thiazolidinediones	Pioglitazone
Dipeptidyl peptidase (DPP) IV inhibitors	Vildagliptin, sitagliptin, saxagliptin, linagliptin
Sodium-glucose cotransporter 2 (SGLT-2) inhibitors	Canagliflozin, dapagliflozin, empagliflozin

Monotherapy	
	Sulfonylurea/Metformin/Thiazolidinediones/DPP IV inhibitors
Dual therapy	
	Sulfonylurea + Metformin
	Sulfonylurea + Thiazolidinedione
	Sulfonylurea + DPP IV inhibitor
	Metformin + Thiazolidinedione
	Metformin + DPP IV inhibitor

Contd...

Contd...

Triple therapy	
	Sulfonylurea + Metformin + Thiazolidinedione
	Metformin + Thiazolidinedione + DPP IV inhibitor

INDICATIONS FOR STARTING INSULIN

- Type 1 diabetes
- Type 2 diabetes—failed treatment with maximal oral antidiabetic drugs (OADs)
- Gestational diabetes
- Stress situations—surgery, infections, acute illness
- Progressive retinopathy, severe neuropathy
- Diabetic ketoacidosis/hyperosmolar hyperglycemic state
- Secondary diabetes—due to pancreatitis/corticosteroids
- Chronic renal failure

CLASSIFICATION OF INSULINS

Type	Duration of action
Short acting insulins	
Aspart	4–6 hr
Lispro	4–6 hr
Glulusine	4 hr
Regular	6–10 hr
Basal insulins	
NPH	14–18 hr
Lente	16–20 hr
Detemir	20 hr
Glargine	24 hr
Degludec	>42 hr
Premixed insulins	
25/75, 30/70, 50/50	

Glucagon-like peptide (GLP-1) analogs
- Exenatide - Liraglutide - Lixisenatide - Dulaglutide
Amylin mimetic
- Pramlintide

Starting Dose for Rapid-acting Insulin[3]

Body weight (kg) × 0.2 divided equally for the 3 meals
[For patients with underlying insulin resistance body weight (kg) × 0.5].

Starting Dose for Basal Bolus Insulin

Body weight (kg) × 0.2
[For patients with underlying insulin resistance body weight (kg) × 0.5].

Correction Factor

3000/kg body weight (or) 1700/total daily dose of insulin (TDD).

For Patients on Tube Feeds[3]

- Basal insulin (glargine once daily or NPH twice daily), TDD 0.3-0.6 unit/kg
- Add a correction dose every 6 hours if using regular insulin or every 4 hours if using analog insulin.

For Patients on Total Parenteral Nutrition

- The target blood glucose level should range between 140-180 mg/dL for critically ill patients and 100-180 mg/dL for stable patients.
- Start with 0.1 unit of regular insulin per gram of carbohydrate in total parenterl nutrition (TPN).
- Monitor blood glucose every 4-6 hours.
- Add a correction dose every 6 hours if using regular insulin or every 4 hours if using analog insulin.

MANAGEMENT OF DIABETIC CARDIOVASCULAR DISEASE[1]

Risk factors include:
- Hypertension
- Hyperglycemia
- Dyslipidemia
- Microalbuminuria
- Smoking.

Blood pressure lowering reduces the risk of both macrovascular and microvascular disease in patients with diabetes. The target blood pressure in these patients should be systole < 140 mm Hg and diastole ≤ 90 mm Hg. These patients can be commenced on
- An ACE inhibitor/ARB or
- Calcium channel blocker or
- A thiazide diuretic.

Beta blockers are indicated in patients with underlying ischemic heart disease and cardiac failure.

Statins are recommended for primary prevention in all type 1 and type 2 diabetics over the age of 40 years regardless of their baseline cholesterol levels.

Intensive lipid lowering therapy with atorvastatin 80 mg OD should be considered for all patients following acute coronary syndromes and revascularization procedures.

Aspirin is not indicated in primary prevention in patients with diabetes. Low-dose aspirin (75 mg) should only be prescribed for patients with proven ischemic heart disease.

MANAGEMENT OF DIABETIC KIDNEY DISEASE[1]

Initially screen for overt proteinuria with urine dip stick. If negative, check urine albumin/creatinine ratio to rule out microalbuminuria.

Periodically monitor the estimated glomerular filtration rate (eGFR).

Microalbuminuria	Urine albumin excretion ranging between 30–300 mg/day or	
	Urine albumin/creatinine ratio (ACR)	
	Men	>2.5 mg/mmol
	Women	>3.5 mg/mmol
Nephropathy	Urine albumin excretion	>300 mg/day
	Urine albumin/creatinine ratio	>30 mg/mmol

Classification of Chronic Kidney Disease

Stage	GFR (mL/min/1.73 m^2)
1	≥90
2	60–89
3A	45–59
3B	30–44
4	15–29
5	<15
5D	On dialysis

Patients with diabetes should be screened annually for diabetic nephropathy from the age of 12 years.

Treatment

- Tight blood sugar control.
- Blood pressure should be reduced to the lowest achievable level.
  - Irrespective of blood pressure, patients with type 1 diabetes and microalbuminuria should receive ACE inhibitors.
  - Irrespective of blood pressure, patients with type 2 diabetes and microalbuminuria should receive either ACE inhibitors or aldosterone receptor blockers (ARBs).

- Patients with chronic kidney disease and proteinuria should be treated with ACE inhibitors or ARBs.
- Statins.
- Management of complications—anemia, renal bone disease, metabolic acidosis.

DIABETIC RETINOPATHY[1]

Screening

- Patients with type 1 diabetes should be screened from 12 years of age.
- Patients with type 2 diabetes should be screened at diagnosis and those with diabetic retinopathy should be screened annually and others once in 2 years.

Risk Factors

- Poor glycemic control
- Hypertension
- Duration of diabetes
- Microalbuminuria and proteinuria
- Pregnancy
- Dyslipidemia.

Good glycemic control (HbA1c around 7%) and good control of blood pressure should be maintained to prevent the onset and progression of diabetic eye disease.

Indications for Laser Photocoagulation

- All patients with type 1 and type 2 diabetes with new vessels at the disc or iris
- All patients with new vessels elsewhere with vitreous hemorrhage
- All patients with type 1 and type 2 diabetes and new vessels elsewhere
- Patients with severe nonproliferative diabetic retinopathy
- Patients with clinically significant macular edema.

DIABETIC FOOT

- These patients should be referred to a multidisciplinary foot clinic.
- Patients with an infected diabetic foot ulcer or underlying osteomyelitis should be commenced on appropriate antibiotics.
- MRI scan is useful in detecting early changes due to Charcot's arthropathy.

DIABETIC PERIPHERAL NEUROPATHY

Assessment	
Small fiber function	Pinprick and temperature
Large fiber function	Vibration, 10 g monofilament, ankle jerk
Protective sensation	10 g monofilament

Treatment of painful neuropathy:
- Antidepressants—tricyclics, duloxetine, venlafaxine
- Anticonvulsants—pregabalin, gabapentin
- Opiate analgesics.

DIABETES IN PREGNANCY[1,4]

Overt diabetes is diagnosed at the first antenatal visit if:
- Random plasma glucose > 200 mg/dL
- Fasting plasma glucose > 126 mg/dL
- HbA1c > 6.5%.

Gestational diabetes mellitus (GDM) is diagnosed between 24–28 weeks of gestation or anytime during pregnancy, if there is an abnormality in the 75 g oral glucose tolerance test (OGTT).

Various professional bodies have used their own criterion to define GDM using the 75 g GTT			
	WHO*	IADPSG** / ADA***	DIPSI****
Fasting	≥126	≥92	Not required
1 hr post-glucose	Not required	≥180	Not required
2-hr post-glucose	≥140	≥153	≥140

*WHO–World Health Organization
**IADPSG-International Association of Diabetes and Pregnancy Study Group
***ADA–American Diabetic Association
****DIPSI-Diabetes in Pregnancy Study Group India

Preconception targets for patients with pre-existing type 1 and type 2 diabetes	
Fasting and premeal plasma glucose	80–110 mg/dL
2-hr postprandial plasma glucose	<155 mg/dL
HbA1c	<6.5%
Comprehensive eye examination	

Metformin or glyburide (Daonil) may be considered as initial treatment for women with gestational diabetes.

Angiotensin converting enzyme (ACE) inhibitors and ARBs are contraindicated during pregnancy. Alpha methyldopa, labetalol and nifedipine can be used for control of blood pressure.

Blood sugar targets during pregnancy	
Premeal	≤95 mg/dL
1 hr postmeal	<140 mg/dL
2-hr postmeal	<120 mg/dL

Blood pressure targets during pregnancy	
Systolic BP	110–129 mm Hg
Diastolic BP	65–79 mm Hg

For patients with both type 1 and type 2 diabetes, retinal examination should be performed prior to conception and during each trimester of pregnancy.

For patients with gestational diabetes GTT with 75 g glucose should be performed 6 weeks after delivery to rule out persisting diabetes.

HYPOGLYCEMIA

Risk Factors
- Long history of diabetes
- HbA1c < 6%
- Autonomic neuropathy
- Patients on insulin and insulin secretagogues
- Older age group.

Treatment
- For conscious patients: Glucose and sugar containing beverages, milk, candy bars and fruit can be used.
- For patients with altered sensorium:
    - 50 mL of 50% dextrose IV followed by an infusion of 5% or 10% dextrose.
    - Inj. glucagon 1 mg IM or SC for nonresponsive patients.

DIABETIC KETOACIDOSIS (DKA)[3,5]

Definition
- Blood glucose > 250 mg/dL
- Metabolic acidosis
    - Arterial pH < 7.3
    - Anion gap > 12
- Positive ketones

Classification	Mild	Moderate	Severe
Venous pH	<7.3	<7.2	<7.1
Bicarbonate (mmol/L)	<15	<10	<5

Treatment

- IV fluids—initially start with normal saline.
  - Administer 1 L over the first 30 minutes.
  - Followed by 1 L over the next 1 hour.
  - Followed by 1 L over the next 2 hours.
  - Subsequently administer 1 L 4 hourly, depending on the degree of dehydration and the central venous pressure (CVP).
- Administer regular insulin 10 units *stat*.
- Start insulin infusion using the formula
  - [Units/hr = (Current blood glucose − 60) × 0.02]
  - If blood glucose is >180 mg/dL multiply by 0.03
  - If blood glucose is <140 mg/dL multiply by 0.01.
- Once the blood glucose drops below 250 mg/dL, switch to 5% dextrose infusion.
- *Potassium*: Do not administer potassium if the patient is anuric or if the potassium is > 5.5 mEq/L.

Serum potassium (mEq/L)	Infusion rate
>5.5	Do not give potassium, repeat potassium after 2 hr
4.5–5.5	10 mEq/L
3.5–4.4	20 mEq/L
<3.5	40 mEq/L and *hold insulin*

- Bicarbonate
  - If arterial pH is <7 give 50 mEq of sodium bicarbonate over 45 minutes.
  - Check blood gas after 30 minute and repeat if pH is <7.
  - Bicarbonate should not be administered if potassium is <3.5 mEq.
- *Phosphate:* If the serum phosphate is <1.0 mg/dL, give 20-30 mEq potassium or sodium phosphate in 1 L of IV fluid.
- When oral fluids are tolerated, IV fluids should be reduced and switch to SC insulin. To prevent rebound hyper glycemia the insulin infusion should overlap the first dose of SC insulin by 30 minutes.

Warning Symptoms and Signs of Cerebral Edema

- Headache and slowing of heart rate.
- Change in neurological status.
- Specific neurological signs.
- Increased blood pressure.
- Decreased oxygen saturation.

Treatment of Cerebral Edema
- Transfer to the ICU
- Restrict IV fluids to 2/3rds of the maintenance dose and give it over 72 hours instead of 24 hours
- Give 20% mannitol 2.5 mL/kg over 20 minutes and repeat after 6 hours
- If there is no response to mannitol give 3% saline 5-10 mL/kg over 30 minutes
- The patient may need intubation.

HYPEROSMOLAR HYPERGLYCEMIC STATE (HHS)[3]

Definition
- Blood glucose > 600 mg/dL
- Serum osmolarity > 320 mOsmol/kg.
- No acidosis or ketones.

Treatment
- Treatment is similar to that of patients with DKA.
- These patients however require more IV fluids and lesser insulin.
- All elderly patients will need a central line and close monitoring of their cardiovascular status.

Monitoring Sheet for Patients with DKA and HHS

Date: Hour:	1	2	3	4	5	6
General condition:						
GCS						
Temperature						
Pulse						
Respiratory rate						
Blood pressure						
Blood glucose (mg/dL)						
Urine ketones						
Electrolytes:						
Sodium (mEq/L)						
Potassium (mEq/L)						
Bicarbonate (mEq/L)						
Blood gas: (arterial/venous)						
pH						
PaO$_2$						
PaCO$_2$						
Insulin:						
IV (units/hour)						
SC (units)						
IV fluids:						

Contd...

Contd...

0.45% saline (mL/hr)					
9% saline (mL/hr)					
5% dextrose (mL/hr)					
Potassium chloride (mEq/hr)					
Oral fluids					
Urine output (mL)					

INSULIN INFUSION[6]

Draw up 40 units of regular insulin and mix it with 39 mL of normal saline, use a syringe pump to deliver 1 unit/mL insulin.

Sliding Scale

RBS (mg/dL)	Insulin infusion rate (mL/hr)
<80	No insulin
81–150	0.5
151–200	1.0
201–250	1.5
251–300	2
301–350	2.5
351–400	3.0
401–450	4.0
451–500	5.0
>500	6

REFERENCES

1. American Diabetes Association. Standards of medical care in diabetes—2018. Diabetes Care. 2018;41(Suppl 1):555-64.
2. Microsoft Word - BGC guideline FINAL - Aug 2009 5 30.doc - di19-diabetes-blood-glucose-control.pdf [Internet]. [Cited 2015 Jan 9]. Available from: http://www.nhmrc.gov.au/_files_nhmrc/file/publications/synopses/di19-diabetes-blood-glucose-control.pdf.
3. Joslin/Beth Israel Deaconess Medical Center - unc_gluc_in_hosp_guideline_final_5_13.pdf [Internet]. [Cited 2015 Jan 9]. Available from: https://www.joslin.org/docs/unc_gluc_in_hosp_guideline_final_5_13.pdf
4. Joslin Diabetes Center and Joslin Clinic, Inc - Preg_guideline_5_10_11_(2)-0615-11.pdf [Internet]. [Cited 2015 Jan 9]. Available from: https://www.joslin.org/bin_from_cms/Preg_guideline_5_10_11_(2)-0615-11.pdf
5. Kitabchi AE, Umpierrez GE, Miles JM, et al. Hyperglycaemic crises in adult patients with diabetes. Diabetes Care. 2009;32(7):1335-43.
6. Magaji V, Johnston JM. Inpatient management of hyperglycemia and diabetes. Clin Diabetes. 2011;29(1):3-9.

CHAPTER 7

Common Calculations and Scoring Systems

MEAN ARTERIAL PRESSURE

$1/3 \times SBP + 2/3 \times DBP$.

LDL CHOLESTEROL

Total cholesterol—HDL - (TG/5).

IDEAL BODY WEIGHT (kg) [AUSTRALIAN MEDICAL HANDBOOK 2014]

- Females = 45.5 kg + 0.9 kg/cm for each cm >152 cm
- Males = 50 kg + 0.9 kg/cm for each cm >152 cm
- Add 10% for heavy frame
- Subtract 10% for light frame.

BODY MASS INDEX (BMI) (kg/m²)

Weight (kg)/height (m^2).

Interpretation

BMI	
<18.5	Below normal weight
18.5–24.9	Normal weight
25–29.9	Overweight
30–34.9	Class I obesity
35–39.9	Class II obesity
>40	Class III obesity

Body Surface Area (The Mosteller Formula)

$[\text{Height (cm)} \times \text{Weight (kg)}/3600]^{1/2}$.

Waist Hip Ratio
- Smallest area around waist/widest area around hip
- Male < 0.85; female < 0.75.

Central Obesity (Waist Circumference)
- Male > 90 cm
- Female > 80 cm.

Basal Energy Expenditure or Basal Metabolic Rate
- Men = 66.5 + [13.75 × Wt (kg) + 5.003 × Ht (cm)] − (Age × 6.775)
- Women = 655.1 + [9.563 × Wt (kg) + 1.850 × Ht (cm)] − (Age × 4.676)

The basal energy expenditure or basal metabolic rate (BEE or BMR) must be multiplied by activity and stress factors to calculate the total caloric requirement.

Calorie Requirement/Day

	Kcal requirement
Little or no exercise	BMR × 1.2
Light exercise (1–3 days per week)	BMR × 1.375
Moderate exercise (3–5 days per week)	BMR × 1.55
Heavy exercise (6–7 days per week)	BMR × 1.725
Very heavy exercise (twice daily or extra heavy workouts)	BMR × 1.9

EASIER METHOD

Considering a resting energy expenditure of 1 kcal/hr/kg of ideal body weight (IBW) in a sedentary individual, 24 kcal will be requirement in a day. If 6 Kcal is added for sedentary work he will require (24 +6) = 30 kcal/kg/day.

Anion Gap
- Na − (Cl + HCO_3^-).
- Normal <11 mEq/L.

ACRONYMS TO REMEMBER THE CAUSES	
Anion Gap Metabolic Acidosis: (MUDPILERS)	*Non-Anion Gap Acidosis:* (HARDUPS)
M: Methanol U: Uremia D: Diabetic or alcoholic ketoacidosis P: Paraldehyde I: Isoniazid L: Lactic acidosis E: Ethylene glycol R: Renal failure S: Salicylates	H: Hyper alimentation A: Acetazolamide R: Renal tubular acidosis D: Diarrhea U: Ureteropelvic shunt P: Post-hypocapnia S: Spironolactone

BICARBONATE DEFICIT

$0.4 \times \text{Wt (kg)} \times (24 - HCO_3)$.

GLUCOSE AND INSULIN

Converting glucose from (mmol to mg): mmol × 18 = mg.
  Estimated average glucose (eAG) from HbA1C: eAG = (28.7 × HbA1C) – 46.7.
  Fasting glucose/insulin <4.5 in patients with polycystic ovary syndrome (PCOS) is consistent with insulin resistance.
  Insulin/glucose ratio >0.3 confirms the diagnosis of hyperinsulism in patients with insulinoma or nesidioblastosis.

HOMA – IR

$$\frac{\text{Fasting insulin (µU/mL)} \times \text{Fasting glucose (mg/dL)}}{405}$$

Serum Osmolality

Serum osmolality = 2 (Na + K) + (BUN/2.8) + (glucose (mg/dL)/18)
  (Or) = 2 (Na + K) + Urea + Glucose (mmol/L)

Sodium Correction for Hyperglycemia

Corrected sodium (Katz, 1973) = Measured sodium + 0.016 × (Serum glucose – 100)

Calcium Correction

Corrected calcium = Serum calcium + 0.8 × (normal albumin-patient's albumin).

Creatinine Clearance

Cockcroft-Gault formula:

$$\text{Male: } \frac{\text{Ideal body weight} \times (140 - \text{Age})}{\text{Serum creatinine} \times 72}$$

$$\text{Female: } \frac{0.85 \times \text{Ideal body weight} \times (140 - \text{Age})}{\text{Serum creatinine} \times 72}$$

Modification of Diet in Renal Disease (MDRD) study equation:
GFR (mL/min/1.73 m²) = $175 \times (S_{cr})^{-1.154} \times (\text{Age})^{-0.203} \times (0.742 \text{ if female}) \times (1.212 \text{ if African American})$

Interpretation

Stage of CKD	eGFR
1	>90
2	60–89

Contd...

Contd...

Stage of CKD	eGFR
3a	45–59
3b	30–44
4	16–29
5	<15 or on dialysis

Fractional Excretion of Sodium (FeNa)

(Plasma creatinine × Urine sodium)/(Plasma sodium × urine creatinine) %

Interpretation

	Prerenal	Intrinsic renal	Postrenal
FE_{Na}	<1%	>1%	>4%
U_{Na} (mmol/L)	<20	>40	>40

Fractional Excretion of Potassium [FeK]

(Urine K × serum Cr × 100)/(Serum K × Urine Cr).

Interpretation

- FeK <10%: Renal cause of hyperkalemia
- FeK >10%: Extrarenal cause of hyperkalemia.

Fractional Excretion of Bicarbonate [$FeHCO_3$]

(Urine HCO_3 × serum Cr)/(Serum HCO_3 × Urine Cr).

Interpretation

- $FeHCO_3$ <5%: Distal RTA
- $FeHCO_3$ >15%: Proximal RTA
- Assumes serum bicarbonate >20 mEq/L.

RENAL TUBULAR REABSORPTION OF PHOSPHATE (TMP/GFR) OR BIJOVET INDEX

1. Calculate the fractional tubular reabsorption of phosphate (TRP):
   TRP = 1 − [(Urinary PO_4/Serum PO_4) × (Serum creatinine/Urinary creatinine)]
2. Plot the serum phosphate and the TRP value on the Bijovet normogram, the intersection of a straight line joining these values gives the TmP/GFR.
   Or
   If the TRP is 0.86 or less then: TMP/GFR = TRP × Serum PO_4
   If the TRP is > 0.86 then: TMP/GFR = 0.3 × TRP / [1 − (0.8 × TRP)] × Serum PO_4

ALDOSTERONE: RENIN RATIO (TO CONFIRM PRIMARY HYPERALDOSTERONISM)

PAC (ng/dL)/PRA (ng/mL/h) >30
(Or)
PAC (ng/dL)/DRC (mU/L) > 3.7
PAC = Plasma aldosterone concentration (ng/dL)
PRA = Plasma renin activity is expressed as (ng/mL/h)
DRC = Direct renin concentration (mU/L) or (ng/L)
Normal aldosterone renin ratio [ARR] cut off based on the assay

	Plasma renin activity [PRA] (ng/mL × hour)	Direct renin concentration [DRC] (mU/L)	Direct renin concentration [DRC] (ng/L)
Plasma aldosterone concentration [PAC] (ng/dL)	30	3.7	5.7

MISCELLANEOUS

Growth Hormone

IU × 0.333 = mg
mg × 3 = IU.

CT scan

An adrenal mass <10 Hounsfield units (HU) suggests an adrenal adenoma. >50% washout after IV contrast, suggests a benign lesion.

Classification of Osteoporosis

	T score
Normal	≥−1.0
Osteopenia	−1 to −2.5
Osteoporosis	≤−2.5
Severe osteoporosis	≤−2.5 with fragility fractures

Thyroid Image Reporting and Data System (TIRADS)

Score	Diagnosis
1	Normal thyroid gland
2	Benign lesions
3	Probably benign lesions
4	Suspicious lesions
	Subclassified as 4a, 4b and 4c
5	Probably malignant lesions
6	Biopsy proven malignancy

THE BETHESDA SYSTEM FOR REPORTING THYROID CYTOPATHOLOGY

Category	Diagnosis	Risk of malignancy
I	Nondiagnostic or unsatisfactory	1–4
II	Benign	0–3
III	Atypia of undetermined significance or follicular lesion of undetermined significance	5–15
IV	Follicular neoplasm or suspicious for a follicular neoplasm	15–30
V	Suspicious for malignancy	60–75
VI	Malignant	97–99

RACPATH CLASSIFICATION OF THYROID FNAC

Thy 1	Nondiagnostic	
	Thy 1c	Cystic lesion
Thy 2	Non-neoplastic	
Thy 3	Possible neoplasm	
	Thy 3a	Atypia
	Thy 3f	Follicular
Thy 4	Suspicious of malignancy	
Thy 5	Malignant	

NO SPECS GRADING OF GRAVES' OPHTHALMOPATHY

Class	Grading
0	No physical signs or symptoms
I	Only signs
II	Soft tissue involvement
III	Proptosis
IV	Extraocular muscle involvement
V	Corneal involvement
VI	Sight loss

CLINICAL ACTIVITY SCORE (CAS) FOR GRAVES' OPHTHALMOPATHY

Clinical parameter	Points
Spontaneous orbital pain	
Gaze evoked orbital pain	

Contd...

Contd...

Clinical parameter	Points
Eyelid swelling	
Eyelid erythema	
Conjunctival redness	
Chemosis	
Inflammation of caruncle	
Total points	

One point is given for each parameter. A score above 3/7 indicates active Graves' ophthalmopathy.

CHAPTER 8

Drug Doses

ANTIEPILEPTICS				
Drugs	Dose	Maximum daily dose	Dose adjustment in renal failure	Route
Carbamazepine	Initial dose: 200 mg BD. Maintenance dose: 800–1200 mg/day		Data not available	PO
Gabapentin	100–300 mg	3600 mg	eGFR <15 mL/min reduce to 300 mg A/D	PO
Lamotrigine	Dosing depends on concomitant antiepileptic medication			
Levetiracetam	Initial dose: 500 mg BD	3000 mg		PO, IV
Oxcarbazepine	Initial dose: 300 mg BD Maintenance dose: 300–1200 mg BD	2400 mg	CrCl ≤ 29 mL/min Initial dose: 150 mg BD	PO
Phenobarbitone	Loading dose: 20 mg/kg IV Maintenance dose: 300 mg/day		eGFR <15 mL/min reduce to 50%	PO, IM, IV
Phenytoin	Loading dose: 15–20 mg/kg (not to exceed 50 mg/min) Maintenance dose: 100 mg TID IV/PO		Nil	PO, IM, IV

Contd...

Contd...

Drugs	Dose	Maximum daily dose	Dose adjustment in renal failure	Route
Pregabalin	75–300 mg/day	300 mg	eGFR 30–60 mL/min 75 mg OD; eGFR 15–30 mL/min 50 mg OD; eGFR <15 mL/min 25 mg OD	PO
Sodium valproate	Initial dose: 10–15 mg/kg IV/PO Maintenance dose: 10–60 mg/kg/day	60 mg/kg	Data not available	PO, IV
Topiramate	Initial dose: 25 mg BD	400 mg	CrCl < 70 mL/min Reduce by 50%	PO
ANTIHYPERTENSIVES				
Amiloride	5 mg OD	10 mg	If CrCl 25–80 mL/min decreased dose by 50%	PO
Amlodipine	2.5–10 mg OD	10 mg		PO
Atenolol	Initial dose: 50 OD Maintenance dose: 50–100 mg/day	100 mg	CrCl 15–35 mL/min Maximum dose 50 mg OD	PO
Bisoprolol	5 mg OD	20 mg	CrCl <40 mL/min Initial dose: 2.5 mg OD	PO
Candesartan	4 mg OD	32 mg	Avoid if eGFR <30 mL/min	PO
Carvedilol	Initial dose: 3.125 mg BD	50–100 mg (depending on the weight)	Stop if renal function worsens	PO
Cilnidipine	5–10 mg	20 mg		PO
Clonidine	Initial dose: 0.1 mg BD	2.4 mg	Lower doses are recommended	PO
Diltiazem	120–240 mg OD	540 mg	Nil	PO, IV

Contd...

Contd...

Drugs	Dose	Maximum daily dose	Dose adjustment in renal failure	Route
Enalapril	5 mg OD	40 mg	CrCl <30 mL/min Initial dose 2.5 mg OD	PO, IV
Eplerenone	25 mg OD	50 mg	Avoid if CrCl is <50 mL/min	PO
Furosemide	20–80 mg	600 mg	Nil	PO, IV
Hydralazine	Initial dose: 10–20 mg QID	300 mg	Nil	PO, IV, IM
	for hypertensive crisis: 20–40 mg IM/IV, repeat as needed			
Hydrochloro-thiazide	25 mg OD	100 mg	Avoid if CrCl is <30 mL/min	PO
Irbesartan	150 mg OD	300 mg	Nil	PO
Labetalol	Initial dose: 100 mg BD. Maintenance dose: 200–400 mg BD.	2400 mg	Nil	PO, IV
Lisinopril	5–10 mg OD	80 mg	CrCl <30 mL/min reduce initial dose by half	PO
Losartan	25–50 mg OD	100 mg	Nil	PO
Methyldopa	Initial dose: 250 mg BD/TID	3 g daily	CrCl 15–50 mL/min The dosage interval should be 8–12 hrs. CrCl <15 mL/min: The dosage interval should be 12–24 hrs.	PO
Metoprolol	Initial dose: 100 mg OD	200 mg	Nil	PO
Nebivolol	5–40 mg/day	40 mg	CrCl <30 mL/min Initial dose: 2.5 mg OD	PO
Nifedipine	10 mg TID	180	Data not available	PO

Contd...

Contd...

Drugs	Dose	Maximum daily dose	Dose adjustment in renal failure	Route
Olmesartan	20 mg	40 mg	Nil	PO
Phenoxy-benzamine	10 mg BD	120 mg		PO
Prazosin	Initial dose: 2–3 mg/day Maintenance dose: 6–15 mg/day	20 mg		PO
Propranolol	Initial dose: 40 mg BD Maintenance dose: 120–240 mg/day	640 mg	Nil	PO
Ramipril	2.5–20 mg	20 mg	CrCl ≤40 mL/min reduce dose by 25%	PO
Sodium nitroprusside	0.5 to 4 µg/kg/min	10 µg/kg/min	Nil	IV
Spironolactone	25–200 mg/day	200 mg	Avoid if eGFR <30 mL/min or creatinine >1.5 mg/dL	PO
Telmisartan	20–80 mg OD	80 mg	Nil	PO
Torsemide	10–20 mg	200 mg	Data not available	PO, IV
Valsartan	Initial dose: 80–160 mg OD	320 mg	Avoid if CrCl is <30 mL/min	PO
Verapamil	180 mg/day	480 mg	Use with caution	PO, IV
ANTI-DIABETIC				
Acarbose	25 mg TID	300 mg	Avoid if serum creatinine > 2 mg/dL	PO
Canagliflozin	100 mg OD	300 mg	Avoid if eGFR< 45 mL/min	PO
Dapagliflozin	5 mg OD	10 mg	Avoid if eGFR< 60 mL/min	PO

Contd...

Contd...

Drugs	Dose	Maximum daily dose	Dose adjustment in renal failure	Route
Dulaglutide	0.75 mg SC once weekly	1.5 mg/week	Nil	SC
Empagliflozin	10 mg OD	25 mg	Avoid if eGFR <45 mL/min	PO
Exenetide	5 µg SC BD	20 µg	Avoid if eGFR <30 mL/min	SC
Glibenclamide	2.5–5 mg	20 mg	Avoid if eGFR <50 mL/min	PO
Gliclazide	40–80 mg	320 mg	Avoid if eGFR <15 mL/min	PO
Glimiperide	1–2 mg	8 mg	Avoid if eGFR <15 mL/min	PO
Glipizide	2.5–5 mg	20 mg	Avoid if eGFR <15 mL/min	PO
Linagliptin	5 mg OD	5 mg		PO
Liraglutide	0.6–1.2 mg SC OD	1.8 mg	Avoid if eGFR <60 mL/min	SC
Lixisenatide	10 µg OD	20 µg	Nil	SC
Metformin	500–1000 mg	2500–3000 mg	Avoid if eGFR <45 mL/min (or) creatinine >1.5	PO
Nateglinide	60–120 mg TID		Nil	PO
Pioglitazone	15–30 mg OD	45 mg	Nil	PO
Pramlintide	Initial dose: 15 µg SC TID	180 µg	Nil	SC
Saxagliptin	2.5–5 mg OD	5 mg	Avoid if eGFR <15 mL/min	PO
Sitagliptin	50–100 mg OD	100 mg	Avoid if eGFR <15 mL/min	PO
Teneligliptin	20–40 mg OD	40 mg	Nil	PO
Vildagliptin	50–100 mg OD	100 mg	Avoid if eGFR <15 mL/min	PO
Voglibose	0.2–0.3 mg TID	0.9 mg		PO
HORMONES				
Anastrazole	1 mg OD		Nil	PO
Clomiphene	For ovulation induction: 50–100 mg OD x 5 days	100 mg OD		PO

Contd...

Contd...

Drugs	Dose	Maximum daily dose	Dose adjustment in renal failure	Route
	For oligospermia: 25–100 mg OD			
Cytomel (T3)	25–75 µg/day			PO
Deflazacort	Initially: up to 12 mg daily Maintenance: 3–8 mg daily			PO
Desmopressin	Initial dose: 50 µg PO BD (or) 1–2 µg SC BD (or) 5–40 µg nasal spray BD			PO, SC, intranasal spray, IV
Dexamethasone	Anti-inflammatory Initial dose: 0.75–9 mg/day		Nil	PO, IV, IM
	For cerebral edema Initial dose: 10 mg IV followed by 4 mg Q6H			IV, IM, PO
	For shock Initial dose: 1–6 mg/kg IV Repeat every 2–6 hours			
17β Estradiol	For induction of puberty Initial dose: 5 µg/kg/day, increase every 6 months	20 µg/kg/day		PO
	Post-oophorectomy 1–2 mg OD			
	Post-menopausal symptoms: 0.45–2 mg OD			
Fludrocortisone	50–100 µg/day			PO
FSH	150 IU thrice weekly			SC
Goserelin	3.6 mg SC every 28 days (or) 10.8 mg SC every 12 weeks		Nil	SC
Human chorionic gonadotropin (hCG)	1500 IU SC thrice weekly			SC

Contd...

Contd...

Drugs	Dose	Maximum daily dose	Dose adjustment in renal failure	Route
Hormone replacement therapy	Conjugated estrogen 0.3–0.625 mg + Medroxyprogesterone acetate 2.5–5 mg OD			PO
Hydrocortisone	For acute conditions 50 IV Q 6 H Maintenance dose: 10–12 mg/M^2/day		Nil	IV, PO
Letrozole	2.5 mg OD			PO
Leuprorelin	3.75 mg IM once a month (or) 11.25 mg IM every 3 months			IM
Methyl-prednisolone	For immunosuppression 250–1000 mg IV OD or A/D x 3–5 doses (or) 4–48 mg PO OD			IV, PO
Octreotide LAR	20–40 mg IM once in 4 weeks			IM
Pitressin	For Diabetes Insipidus 5–10 units IM/SC 8–12 hourly (or) Intravenous infusion at the rate of 0.5 mU/kg/hr = 0.1mL/kg/hr			IM, SC, IV
	For Vasodilatory shock 0.01–0.04 units/min IV			IV
Prednisolone	For anti-inflammatory action 5–60 mg/day			PO
	For maintenance 2.5–5 mg OD			
Tamoxifen	20–40 mg/day			PO
Testosterone	For induction of puberty: Testosterone enantate (Sustanon) 50–75 mg/month, increase every 6 months to 100–150 mg/month, after 3 years continue 250 mg once in 3 weeks			
	For maintenance: in adults >18 years of age, Testosterone Undecanoate 1000 mg once every 10–14 weeks			
Dose equivalents: Hydrocortisone 20 mg = Prednisolone 5 mg = Methyl prednisolone 4 mg = Dexamethasone 0.75 mg Methyl prednisolone/0.8 = Prednisolone dose				

Contd...

Contd...

OSTEOPOROSIS

Drugs	Dose	Maximum daily dose	Dose adjustment in renal failure	Route
Alendronate	10 mg OD (or) 70 mg once a week		Avoid	PO
Calcitonin	For osteoporosis 50–400 IU SC OD			SC, IM, Intranasal
	For hypercalcemia 4 IU/kg Q12H			
Calcium	Supplements 500–600 mg BD		Data not available	
	For severe hypocalcemia: ~3 g Calcium gluconate IV over 5–10 minutes followed by continuous infusion 0.5–2 mg/kg/hr			
Calcitriol	0.25 µg OD; increasing upto 0.5 µg BD, if required	1µg	Nil	PO
Cinacalcet	30 mg OD	360 mg	Nil	PO
Denosumab	For osteoporosis: 60 mg SC once in 6 months		Nil	SC
	For other indications: 120 mg once in 4 weeks			
Ibandronate	2.5 mg OD (or) 150 mg once a month		Avoid	PO
Pamidronate	60–90 mg given as a slow infusion over 4 hours once in 3–4 weeks	90 mg		IV
Teriparatide	20 µg SC OD			SC
Vitamin D			Nil	PO, IM
For levels <20 ng/mL	50–60,000 units once a week for 6–8 weeks, followed by 50–60,000 units once a month			
20–30 ng/mL	50–60,000 units once a month			
Zolindronic acid	4 mg as a slow infusion, once a year		Avoid	IV
MISCELLANEOUS				
Amitriptyline	25 mg HS	300 mg	Nil	PO

Contd...

Contd...

Drugs	Dose	Maximum daily dose	Dose adjustment in renal failure	Route
Diazoxide	For hypoglycemia: 3–8 mg/kg/day	15 mg/kg/day		PO
	For hypertensive emergency: 1–3 mg/kg (maximum 150 mg) every 5–15 minutes, then every 4–24 hours			IV
Enoxaparin	1.5 mg/kg OD (or) 1 mg/kg SC BD			SC
Fondaparinux				SC
Weight <50 kg	5 mg SC OD			
50–100 kg	7.5 mg SC OD			
>100 kg	10 mg SC OD			
Heparin	80 units/kg bolus, followed by 18 units/kg/hr as infusion, adjust the dose according to aPTT			
Methylcobalamine	500 µg TID	1500 µg		PO, IM, IV
Salbutamol			Nil	
	For acute asthma: 2.5 mg 3–4 times a day			Nebulized
	For asthma maintenance: 200 µg every 4–6 hours	800 µg		Inhaler
	For hyperkalemia: 20 mg in 4 mL normal saline solution nebulized over 10 minutes			Nebulized
Sildenafil	For erectile dysfunction: Initial dose 50 mg/day Maintenance dose 25–50 mg/day		If eGFR <30/mL/min 25 mg/day	PO
Tadalafil	Initial dose 10 mg/day; Maintenance dose 5–20 mg/day			
Thiamine	50–100 mg OD	300 mg	Nil	PO, IV, IM

FOR RESUSCITATION			
Drugs	Dose	Route	Rate of infusion
Adrenaline	Concentration (1:10,000) or 0.1 mg/mL In cardiac arrest: 0.5–1 mg (5–10 mL) stat, repeat every 5 minutes if required	IV, IM, SC	0.1–1.5 µg/kg/min
Atropine	In cardiac arrest or bradycardia: 0.6 mg IV stat, repeat every 15 minutes if required	IV, IM, SC, ET	0.02–0.08 mg/kg/hr
Dopamine	For shock: Initial dose 1–5 µg/kg/min, titrate up to 50 µg/kg/min	IV	1–50 µg/kg/min
Dobutamine	For congestive cardiac failure: Initial dose: 0.5–1 µg/kg/min Maintenance dose: 2–20 µg/kg/min	IV	0.5–40 µg/kg/min
Glyceryl trinitrate		IV, sublingual, aerosol spray, transdermal	
	For acute angina: Tablet: 300–600 µg, repeat if necessary Aerosol spray: 400–800 µg		
	For unstable angina: Initial dose 5–15 µg/min		10–200 µg/min
	For hypertensive emergencies: Initial dose 5–25 µg/min		10–200 µg/min
Noradrenaline	Concentration 1mg/mL For hypotension: Initial dose 2–4 µg/min Maintenance dose 1–12 µg/min		1–12 µg/min
Sodium bicarbonate	8.4% (1 mmol/mL)		
	For asystole: Initially 1 mEq/kg, if required repeat 0.5 mEq/kg after 10 minutes		
	For hyperkalemia: 150 mEq in 1 litre D5W over 2–4 hours		
Vasopressin	For asystole, ventricular fibrillation and ventricular tachycardia 40 units IV followed by 20 mL normal saline. If spontaneous circulation is not restored within 3 minutes another 40 units is given IV	IV	

Index

A

Acarbose 46, 66
Acetazolamide 57
Acidosis, metabolic 52
Acromegaly 9, 15
Adrenal gland 6, 25
Adrenal hyperplasia, congenital 18, 26
Adrenal insufficiency 36, 41
    primary 26
    secondary 26
Adrenaline 72
Adrenocorticotropic hormone,
    assessment of 11
Adrogue formula 32
Aldosterone receptor blockers 49
Alendronate 70
Alpha glucosidase inhibitors 46
Amiloride 64
Amitriptyline 70
Amlodipine 64
Anastrazole 67
Androgen excess 7
Angiotensin converting enzyme
    inhibitors 51
Anion gap 57
    metabolic acidosis 57
Anterior pituitary function, assessment
    of 11
Antibody titers 45
Anticoagulation 43
Anticonvulsants 51
Antidepressants 51
Anxiety 42
Arrhythmias 42
    cardiac 27
Arteritis, temporal 43
Atenolol 64
Atropine 72

B

Basal bolus insulin 48
Basal energy expenditure 57
Basal metabolic rate 57
Bethesda system 61
Bicarbonate 52, 53, 58
    fractional excretion of 59
Biguanides 46
Bijovet index 59
Biopsy proven malignancy 60
Bisoprolol 64
Blood
    glucose 52
    pressure 46, 52
    sugar 45, 52
Body mass index 56
Body surface area 56
Bone profile 1, 40
Bradycardia 39
Broad spectrum antibiotic cover 39
Burch-Wartofsky score 37

C

Cabergoline 43
Calcitonin 70
Calcitriol 70
Calcium 70
    correction 58
    infusion test 23
        interpretation 24
        preparation 23
        procedures 23
Canagliflozin 46, 66
Candesartan 64
Carbamazepine 63
Carbimazole 38
Carcinoid tumors 28
Cardiovascular dysfunction 37
Caruncle, inflammation of 62
Carvedilol 64
Cavernous sinus thrombosis 43
Central nervous system disturbance 38
Central venous pressure 53
Cerebral edema
    signs of 53
    treatment of 54

Cerebrovascular
  accidents 42
  seizures 42
Charcot's arthropathy 50
Chemosis 62
Chemotherapy 41
Chromogranin A 28
Chronic kidney disease, classification of 49
Cilnidipine 64
Cinacalcet 70
Clinical biochemistry, reference ranges 1
Clomiphene 67
Clonidine 64
  dose 14
  test 14
    indication 14
    interpretation 14
    precaution 14
    procedures 14
Common calculations and scoring systems 56
Conjunctival redness 62
Corticosteroids 47
Cortisol day curve 21
  indication 21
  interpretation 21
  preparation 21
  procedure 21
Creatinine 40, 43
CRH stimulation test 19
  indication 19
  procedures 19
Cushing's disease 9, 17, 20, 21
Cushing's syndrome 17, 19

D

Dapagliflozin 46, 66
Deflazacort 68
Dehydration 23
Denosumab 70
Desmopressin 68
  test 20, 22
    indication 20
    interpretation 21
    procedures 21
DEXA-CRH test 19
  indication 19
  interpretations 19
  procedures 19
Dexamethasone 68, 69
Diabetes
  duration of 50
  insipidus 10, 43
  mellitus 5, 45
    gestational 47, 51
    protocols 45
    secondary 47
    type 1 47
    type 2 47
Diabetic cardiovascular disease, management of 48
Diabetic foot 50
Diabetic kidney disease, management of 49
Diarrhea 38, 57
Diazoxide 71
Dihydrotestosterone 28
Diltiazem 64
Dipeptidyl peptidase IV inhibitors 46
Dobutamine 72
Dopamine 72
Drugs 63-72
Dulaglutide 67
Duloxetine 51
Dyslipidemia 48, 50

E

Edema
  pedal 38
  pulmonary 38, 42
Empagliflozin 46, 67
Enalapril 65
Encephalopathy, hypertensive 43
Endocrine
  disorders, evaluation of 4
  emergencies 37
  test protocols 11
Enoxaparin 71
Epilepsy 11
Eplerenone 65
Estradiol 15
Ethylene glycol 57
Exenetide 67
Eyelid
  erythema 62
  swelling 62

F

Fasting glucose 45
Fludrocortisone 68
Follicle-stimulating hormone 15
Fondaparinux 71
Forty eight or seventy two hour fast 24
   indications 24
   interpretations 25
   preparation 24
   procedures 24
Furosemide 65

G

Gabapentin 51, 63
Gastrointestinal dysfunction 38
Gaze evoked orbital pain 61
Glibenclamide 46, 67
Gliclazide 46, 67
Glimiperide 46, 67
Glipizide 46, 67
Glucagon dose 13
Glucagon test 13
   contraindications 13
   indications 13
   procedures 13
Glucocorticoid excess 6
Glucose 58
Glyburide 51
Glycemic criteria 46
Glyceryl trinitrate 72
Gonadal function 15
Gonadotroph adenomas 10
Gonadotropin releasing hormone
   analog dose 15
   therapy 43
Gonadotropin releasing hormone
      analog test 15
   indications 15
   interpretations 15
   procedures 15
Goserelin 68
Graves' ophthalmopathy 61
Growth hormone 16, 60
   reserve, assessment of 11
   status after surgery, assessment of 16

H

Head injury 43
Headache 42
Heart
   disease, ischemic 11
   failure, congestive 38
Hemorrhage
   cerebral 43
   subarachnoid 43
Heparin 71
High-dose dexamethasone suppression
      test 19
   contraindications 19
   interpretations 20
   procedures 20
Hormone 67
   assays 2
   replacement therapy 17
Hounsfield units 60
Human chorionic gonadotropin 68
   stimulation test 27
      indications 27
      interpretations 28
      procedures 28
Hungry bone syndrome 41
Hydralazine 65
Hydrochlorothiazide 65
Hydrocortisone 39, 69
   replacement 36
Hydroxylase deficiency, partial 18
Hyperaldosteronism 27, 60
Hypercalcemia 35, 40
   classification 35
   treatment 35
Hypercortisolemic state, establishing 17
Hyperglycemia 48
   sodium correction for 58
   symptoms of 45
Hyperkalemia 33
   classification 33
   treatment 33
Hypernatremia 32
   calculation 32
   classification 32, 33
   treatment 33
Hyperosmolar hyperglycemic state 47, 54
Hyperphosphatemia 41
Hypertension 48, 50
   uncontrolled 27
Hypertensive crises, treatment of 42
Hypocalcemia 34, 41

classification 34
mild 34
severe 34
Hypoglycemia 39, 52
   classification of 46
   correction of 39
Hypokalemia 33, 35
   classification 33
   mild to moderate 33
   severe 27
   treatment 33
Hypomagnesemia 35, 41
   grading 35
   treatment 35
Hyponatremia 31, 39
   asymptomatic 32
   calculation 31
   classification 31
   postoperative 10
   severe 39
   treatment 32
Hypoparathyroidism 41
Hypopituitarism 11
Hypotension 39
   treatment of 39
Hypothermia 39
Hypothyroidism, severe 11, 13
Hypoventilation 39

I

Ibandronate 70
Impaired fasting glucose 45
Impaired glucose tolerance 45
Infection 37
Inferior petrosal sinus sampling 20
   indication 20
   interpretations 20
   procedures 20
Insulin 58
   classification of 47
   infusion 55
   tolerance test 11, 13
      contraindications 11
      indications 11
Insulinoma 13
Intravenous fluids, sodium content of 32
Irbesartan 65
Isoniazid 57

J

Jaundice 38

K

Ketoacidosis
   alcoholic 57
   diabetic 37, 47, 52, 57

L

Labetalol 65
Lactic acidosis 57
Lamotrigine 63
Laser photocoagulation 50
Letrozole 69
Leuprorelin 69
Levetiracetam 63
Linagliptin 46, 67
Liraglutide 67
Lisinopril 65
Liver
   disease, chronic 13
   function tests 1
Lixisenatide 67
Losartan 65
Low-dose dexamethasone suppression test 18
   contraindications 18
   indications 18
   interpretations 18
   procedures 18
Luteinizing hormone 15

M

Magnesium sulfate 42
Mean arterial pressure 56
Mean growth hormone 16
Medullary thyroid carcinoma 23
Meglitinides 46
Meningitis 43
Metformin 46, 47, 51, 67
Methanol 57
Methylcobalamin 71
Methyldopa 65
Methyl-prednisolone 69
Metoprolol 65
Microalbuminuria 48-50
Monotherapy 46
Mosteller formula 56
Myxedema coma 39

N

Nateglinide 46, 67
Nausea 38, 42

Nebivolol 65
Nephropathy 49
Neuropathy
    diabetic peripheral 51
    severe 47
Nifedipine 65
Night-time salivary cortisol 17
Non-anion gap acidosis 57
Noradrenaline 72

O

Obesity, central 57
Octreotide lar 69
Olmesartan 66
Ophthalmoplegia 42
Opiate analgesics 51
Oral antidiabetic drugs 46
Oral glucose tolerance test 15, 16, 51
    for assessment of diabetic status 24
        interpretation 24
        preparations 24
        procedure 24
    indication 15
    interpretation 16
    precaution 15
    procedures 15
Oral iodine 39
Orbital pain, spontaneous 61
Osteopenia 60
Osteoporosis 60
    classification of 60
    severe 60
Ovary 8
Overnight dexamethasone suppression test 17
    contraindications 17
    interpretation 18
    procedures 18
    indication 17, 18
Oxcarbazepine 63

P

Pain 38
Pamidronate 70
Pancreas 5, 24
Pancreatic neuroendocrine tumors 28
Pancreatitis 41, 47
Paraldehyde 57
Parathyroid 5
    hormone 40
Paresthesia 41

Peak postprandial capillary plasma glucose 45
Peptide analogs, glucagon-like 47
Phenobarbitone 63
Phenoxybenzamine 66
Phenytoin 63
Pheochromocytoma 7, 13, 42
Phosphate 53
    renal tubular reabsorption of 59
Pioglitazone 46, 67
Pitressin 69
Pituitary apoplexy 42
Plasma
    creatinine 59
    sodium 59
Polycystic ovary syndrome 18, 58
Poor glycemic control 50
Potassium, fractional excretion of 59
Pramlintide 67
Prazosin 66
Prediabetes 45
Prednisolone 69
Pregabalin 51, 64
Pregnancy, toxemia of 37
Preprandial capillary plasma glucose 45
Prolactinomas 9
Propranolol 66
Propylthiouracil 38
Proteinuria 50
Pseudo-Cushing's syndrome 19
Puberty
    central precocious 15
    disorders of 15
    peripheral precocious 15

R

Radioiodine therapy 37
Ramipril 66
Random plasma glucose 45
Rapid-acting insulin 47
Renal tubular acidosis 57
Repaglinide 46
Retinopathy
    diabetic 50
    progressive 47

S

Salbutamol 71
Salicylates 57
Saline infusion test 27

contraindications 27
indication 27
interpretations 27
preparations 27
procedures 27
Saxagliptin 46, 67
Seizures 41
Serum electrolytes 40, 43
    creatinine 41
Short synacthen test 25
    indications 25
    interpretations 26
    preparations 25
    procedures 26
Sildenafil 71
Sitagliptin 46, 67
Sliding scale 55
Small fiber function 51
Sodium
    bicarbonate 72
    fractional excretion of 59
    glucose cotransporter 2 46
    nitroprusside 66
        infusion 42
    total body deficit of 31
    valproate 64
Spironolactone 57, 66
Stress situations 47
Sulfonylurea 46, 47
Sweating 42

T

Tachycardia 37
Tadalafil 71
Tamoxifen 69
Telmisartan 66
Teneligliptin 67
Teriparatide 70
Testis 8, 27
Testosterone 15, 28, 69
Tetany 41
Thermoregulatory dysfunction 37
Thiamine 71
Thiazolidinedione 46, 47
Third nerve palsy, diabetic 43
Thyroid 4
    cytopathology 61
    gland, normal 60
    image reporting and data system 60
    malignancy 4
    profile 38
    storm 37
Thyroxine 39
Topiramate 64
Torsemide 66
Total parenteral nutrition 48
Trauma 37
Triglycerides 46
Triple therapy 47
Tube feeds 48
Twenty-four hour urinary free cortisol 17

U

Uremia 57
Ureteropelvic shunt 57
Urine
    creatinine 59
    osmolality 43
    sodium 59

V

Valsartan 66
Vasopressin 72
Venlafaxine 51
Verapamil 66
Vertigo 42
Vildagliptin 46, 67
Visual acuity 42
Vitamin D 40, 70
    deficiency 41
Voglibose 46, 67
Vomiting 38, 42

W

Waist
    circumference 57
    hip ratio 57
Water deprivation test 21, 22
    interpretation 23
    preparations 21
    procedure 22

Z

Zinc transporter 8 islet antibody 45

Printed by Libri Plureos GmbH in Hamburg, Germany